VARICOSE VEINS

Harold Ellis recently retired as Professor of Surgery at Westminster Medical School, University of London. He has specialized in the treatment of varicose veins for thirty years and has run the busy varicose veins clinic at Westminster Hospital since 1962. He was also a member of the Council of the Royal College of Surgeons of England. He now teaches anatomy in Cambridge.

He is well known around the world not only through his frequent lecture tours for the British Council and other organizations, but also for his hundreds of papers on surgical topics and his numerous medical textbooks, including *Clinical Anatomy, Lecture Notes on General Surgery, Maingot's Abdominal Operations* and *Anatomy for Anaesthetists.*

Professor Ellis is married and the father of two children. He lives in north London where his chief leisure interest is medical history. In 1987 he was awarded the CBE.

VARICOSE VEINS

How they are treated, and what you can do to help

Professor Harold Ellis, CBE, MA, DM, FRCS

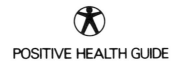

POSITIVE HEALTH GUIDE

© Harold Ellis 1982

Reprinted 1984

First published in the United Kingdom in 1982
by Martin Dunitz Limited, London
This edition published in 1991 by
Macdonald Optima, a division of
Macdonald & Co. (Publishers) Ltd

A member of Maxwell Macmillan
Pergamon Publishing Corporation

British Library Cataloguing in Publication Data
Ellis, Harold 1926–
    Varicose veins.
    1. Man. Veins. Varicose veins
    I. Title   II. Series
    616.143

    ISBN 0–356–19771–9

Macdonald & Co. (Publishers) Ltd
Orbit House
1 New Fetter Lane
London EC4A 1AR

Typeset by Leaper & Gard Limited, Bristol, England
Printed by Toppan Printing Company (S) Pte. Ltd. Singapore

CONTENTS

FOREWORD

Harry S. Goldsmith, MD
Professor of Surgery, Dartmouth Medical School, Hanover, USA

Professor Harold Ellis's well-deserved reputation as one of the finest surgical teachers, both in Britain and throughout the world, has resulted from his captivating lecture style as well as through his many papers and textbooks dealing with surgery. This book on varicose veins is another accomplishment, because he has now expanded with apparent ease his teaching audience from professionals within the medical field to the general public.

Anyone with historical awareness knows that the patient has rarely been given the opportunity to understand the physical nature of his disorder and the range of available therapy. In effect, the medical profession has assumed responsibility for patient care and yet has often been insensitive to the patient's desire to be more aware of the intricacies of his illness. Because Professor Ellis knows that today's patient not only wants but frequently demands to know the fundamentals of his condition, *Varicose Veins* explains in clear terms how the problem develops and how it can be treated. Indeed, all the questions the sufferer is likely to ask are answered in a very full and lucid manner. Professor Ellis is to be congratulated on the clarity with which he has assembled this information for the vast number of patients with varicose veins.

1 THE PROBLEM IN PERSPECTIVE

If you talk to patients sitting in a general surgical out-patient clinic you will find that three problems have brought the vast majority of them there – hernias, piles and, of course, varicose veins. These three conditions share a number of features: they are common, they are embarrassing, they are a nuisance and there is nothing yet known to medical science that will actually prevent any of them.

Unfortunately, therefore, there is absolutely nothing you can do to stop yourself from getting varicose veins, but there are certain things you should know about your varicose veins and quite a number of other things you can do to prevent them from getting worse and to help your doctor to make you better.

Exactly what varicose veins are I shall be describing fully in the next chapter. Most people have a fairly good idea what they look like. Indeed they are probably the commonest reason for people to be admitted to the general surgical departments of hospitals throughout the Western civilized world. In Britain, for instance, one person in five already has or is likely to develop varicose veins to some degree; and women are far more likely to suffer from them than men.

Don't get the wrong idea

Because varicose veins are so common, it is not surprising that many mistaken, even wrong, ideas have developed about them. People with almost the first sign of vein troubles become worried that they may develop the rather nasty complications that seem to lead on from this condition – the brownish-black stain known as pigmentation; the open, slow-to-heal wound of ulceration; thrombosis or clotting; and so on.

As far as these complications go, you can be reassured. In the first place, nothing happens quickly. A small varicose vein on the leg does not suddenly grow into a mass of grape-like structures from ankle to groin. In fact, the time-span is measured in many years. Similarly, if you develop a little patch of eczema or pigmentation on the leg, although you should regard it as a warning that treatment is necessary, it is not suddenly going to turn into a huge varicose ulcer.

If you discover that you have varicose veins developing then do report them to your doctor. It may well be that they will not get any bigger but it is advisable to keep them under observation. They may never need any treatment. When the veins are more marked in otherwise healthy and active people, then they should certainly be treated and this will prevent those unpleasant complications from occurring. If you have old and infirm relatives with varicose veins, their treatment will probably consist only of support stockings which will help to keep the veins under control and the legs comfortable.

It is important to remember that just because you have varicose veins it does not mean that every ache and pain or other symptom in the leg stems from them. See your doctor so that he can check your leg carefully for other problems such as sciatica or arthritis before deciding that the cause is in fact your varicose veins. Also, there may be other blemishes on your skin that you might think are varicose veins but are not varicose veins at all. Your doctor should soon put your mind at rest about these. Some of the more common misconceptions are dealt with in chapter eight.

Treatment

What about removal of varicose veins for cosmetic reasons? Most people like to look their best. Many spend a great deal of time and effort on their appearance, and to some, especially those whose professions keep them in the public eye, the presence of very obvious and discoloured veins in their legs is a real embarrassment. Even if there is no aching or discomfort, there is no reason why the veins should not be dealt with for cosmetic reasons, and indeed, this is one of the most frequent indications for their treatment.

Nevertheless, the treatment and after-care of varicose veins is the same whether it is primarily for health or cosmetic reasons. So, all is not lost just because you have varicose veins; there is much you can do. Here are a number of common-sense tips that may give you the key to a healthy, active life in spite of varicose veins.

Help yourself to healthy legs

Exercise   This will improve the flow of blood in your legs and also help to pump the blood from your legs back to your lungs. Jogging, swimming and cycling are all first-class activities but walking is even better – and a superb exercise that can be carried out by almost anybody at any age. Leave your car in the garage, forget about the bus, avoid the elevator, and walk!

Don't stand around Learn to put your legs up when you are sitting quietly at home and raise your legs in bed at night. This will help the veins to empty and will prevent or reduce any puffiness in your feet. Few people wear tight garters nowadays; but if you do, and you have varicose veins, you should throw the garters away.

Watch your weight The surgeon's heart sinks when he sees a fat patient with varicose veins. He knows that injection treatment is going to be difficult and that the risks of surgery will be increased. You will help him and yourself if you slim down, and you will also look and feel better!

It may be that your veins have already reached the stage of dis-colouration and ulceration. Your surgeon will be able to do a great deal to help you, but afterwards you will have a lifetime's respon-sibility for the care of your legs. This means elastic support, keeping your legs raised at night, active exercises and weight watching. The more vigilant you are, the more remote your chances of a recurrence.

So once the doctor has done his part it is largely up to you to help yourself to get better and to stay cured. As you read through this book you will be taking the first steps to that end.

2 WHAT ARE VARICOSE VEINS?

There are, of course, veins all over our bodies, some deep within the tissues and some, the superficial veins, near the surface of our skin. Like any other organ they too can go wrong and it seems that the veins in our legs are more vulnerable than those almost anywhere else in our blood circulatory system.

What, then, makes an ordinary surface leg vein into a varicose vein? A varicose vein is in fact a vein that has lost its elasticity; it has become weak and flabby and expands, or dilates, easily. The first sign that one of your veins is varicose is that when you stand up the vein becomes obviously swollen with blood. But why, you might

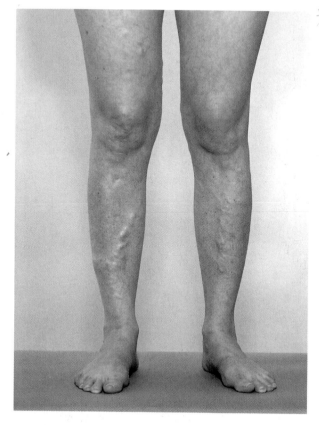

A typical example of varicose veins showing how they swell when you stand up.

ask, should veins become dilated when you stand up? Why is it that only veins become varicose? To answer these questions and to help you understand the underlying causes for your varicose veins we should take a look at the way blood circulates around our bodies and the part veins play in the process.

The circulation of the blood

Most of you will probably need your memories jogged back to schooldays when you did a little anatomy in your biology classes or

The circulation

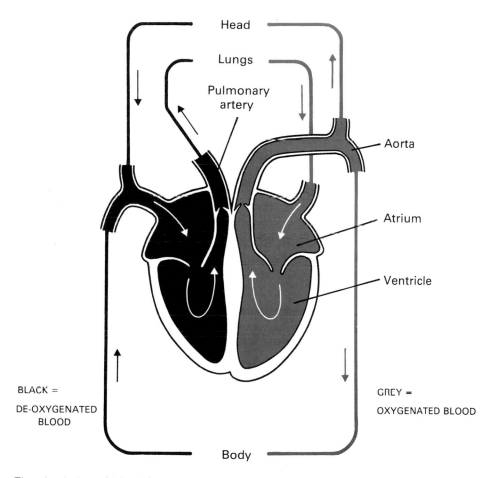

The circulation of blood from the body through the heart to the lungs. From the lungs the oxygenated blood returns to the heart and circulates to the rest of the body.

when you were taught first aid.

The heart itself (see previous page) is really just a muscular pump, roughly the size of your own fist. Actually it's a double pump, divided down the middle into right and left compartments. These compartments are further divided into top and bottom chambers. The top chambers, known as atria, are thin-walled. The bottom chambers, the ventricles, have thick muscular walls.

The left ventricle has the job of pumping out blood all around the body and so has thicker walls than the right ventricle which pumps blood only to the lungs. The right side of the heart receives blood from the veins, whose job it is to return blood from every part of the body (apart from the lungs) to the heart; this blood is then pumped into the lungs. The left side of the heart receives only the blood returning from the lungs and pumps this out into all parts of the body, thus completing the cycle.

The functions of the blood

The blood that enters the right side of the heart from the veins has already given up a good deal of its oxygen to the body's tissues and in turn has received waste products produced by the body, particularly carbon dioxide. This blood is dark blue in colour because it is low in oxygen (which turns blood cells red) and is known as venous, or deoxygenated, blood.

Venous blood – that is to say, blood from the veins – enters the right atrium, passes through a one-way valve and enters the right ventricle. From here the blood is pumped through the pulmonary (or lung) valve, which allows only a one-way flow, into the pulmonary arteries and through them into the lungs. Once in the lungs, the venous blood enters a network of minute hair-like vessels known as capillaries which spread the blood over the surface of the sponge-like lung tissue. The blood gives up the carbon dioxide, which is breathed out in the expired air. Oxygen from the breathed-in air is.meanwhile taken into the blood, which then returns to the left side of the heart into the atrium. From here the blood passes into the left ventricle. This freshly oxygenated blood is then pumped out through the main artery, the aorta, crossing the aortic valve, which prevents the blood flooding back into the heart, for distribution throughout the body.

The heart is one of those structures that amaze both doctors and engineers. It carries out a steady rhythmic activity, contracting about seventy times a minute, year in, year out, often for seventy years or more without any trouble. It pumps about 4,000 gallons (18,200 litres) of blood daily through something like a 60,000-mile (96,500-km) network of blood vessels. It has the ability accurately to adjust its rate and force to your body's needs, increasing during exercise, slowing while you sleep. If any inventor could create a machine anywhere near approaching such simplicity and efficiency the world would be at his feet!

The arteries, capillaries and veins

The muscular pump of the heart is the motive power that drives the blood out into all the main arteries. This driving force in each of us is measured as our blood pressure, which in a healthy young adult is powerful enough to raise a column of mercury about 120 mm high. This is what the doctor measures in millimetres of mercury (mmHg) when he wraps an inflatable cuff around your arm and takes your blood pressure.

The function of the arteries is to distribute oxygenated blood throughout our bodies. Their tough, partly elastic, partly muscular, smooth-walled tubes progressively divide, rather like the branches

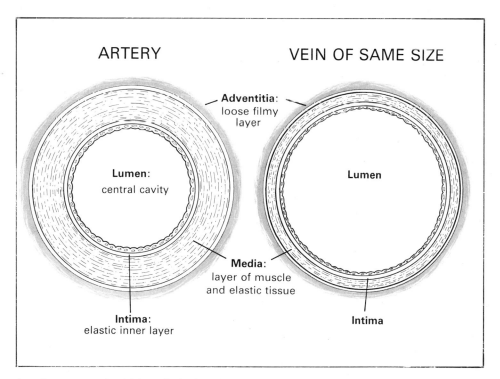

Arteries are tough, thick-walled tubes. Veins are thin and flimsy in comparison, and their lack of muscle makes them susceptible to swelling.

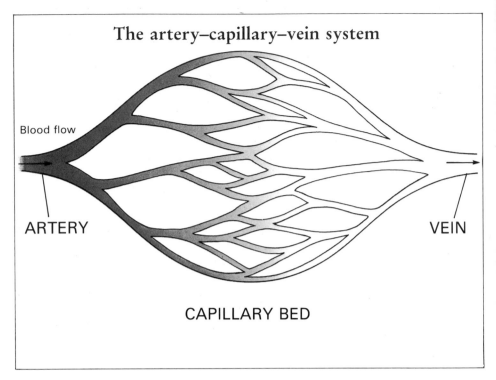

The artery–capillary–vein system

Blood flow

ARTERY

VEIN

CAPILLARY BED

Arteries carry blood to the tiny capillaries where it gives up its oxygen and nutrients. The blood is carried back to the heart by the veins.

of a tree, into smaller and smaller channels down to the capillaries. These minute tubes, the thickness of a single cell, are often only wide enough to allow the blood corpuscles to squeeze along them one at a time. You can get some idea of just how small they are when you realize that blood corpuscles measure only seven-thousandths of a millimetre in diameter.

It is at capillary level that the blood carries out its vital job of nourishing the tissues of our bodies. Oxygen and essential nutrients such as sugar are passed through the capillary walls to the tissues, while carbon dioxide and chemicals such as urea – the waste products of cell activity – pass back into the blood and are eventually passed out of our bodies.

The capillary network then re-forms, first into tiny tubes known as venules, which then join up with each other to form the veins. The veins have only one purpose and that is to carry blood back to the heart. In contrast to the thick-walled, muscular arteries, your veins are thin tubes, mostly made up of supporting connective tissue, and have only small amounts of muscle in their walls.

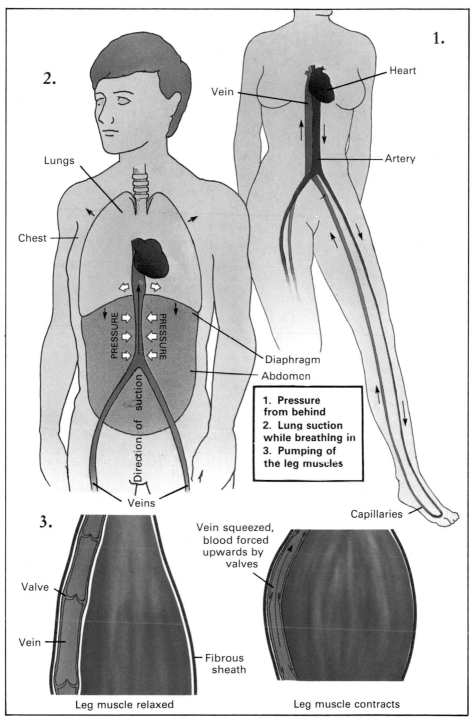

2.

Lungs

Chest

Heart

Vein

Artery

1.

PRESSURE

PRESSURE

Direction of suction

Diaphragm

Abdomen

1. Pressure from behind
2. Lung suction while breathing in
3. Pumping of the leg muscles

Veins

Capillaries

3.

Valve

Vein

Vein squeezed, blood forced upwards by valves

Fibrous sheath

Leg muscle relaxed

Leg muscle contracts

The three forces helping to keep blood moving in the leg veins.

Keeping blood moving in the veins

As the blood trickles through the network of capillaries, the pressure falls to only a few mmHg, so what is the force that gets the blood back along the veins to the heart? When we lie down the force of gravity helps the flow along but what about when we stand up and blood has to be forced uphill from the veins in the feet back to the heart?

There are three things that help (see diagram on previous page). The first is the pressure from behind, the slight pressure pushing blood onwards from the capillaries into the venules. Although this is sufficient when we lie down, it is totally inadequate when we are standing or walking. Second is the suction effect of the lungs; when we take a deep breath a negative pressure rather like a vacuum is created in the chest which helps draw blood upwards to the heart. The third, however, is the most important of all. It is in fact a brilliant mechanism: the pumping action of the leg muscles. These muscles are enclosed in a dense sheath of fibrous tissue (called by doctors the deep fascia). When you walk about, the muscles contract

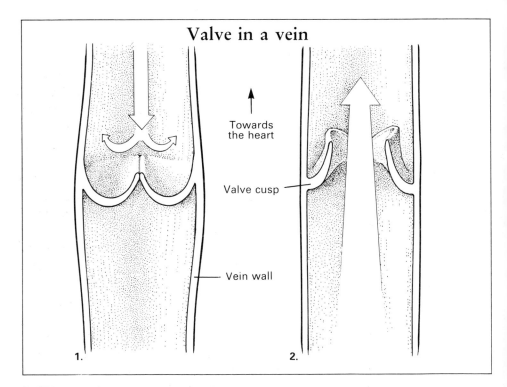

Valve in a vein

Towards the heart

Valve cusp

Vein wall

1.   2.

1. The two valve cusps come together, preventing back flow of blood.   2. These valves only open to allow blood to travel towards the heart.

and the veins contained in the fibrous sheath are squeezed. At intervals along the insides of the veins are beautifully constructed valves, consisting of two flaps that exactly meet each other. Though very simple they are quite sufficient nevertheless to make sure that the blood can be squeezed in one direction only – back to the heart.

Now while all this seems like a clever solution to pump the blood in our veins back to the heart there remains one problem and that is how to get blood back from the skin and the fatty tissues of the leg that lie *outside* this fibrous sheath.

Again, an ingenious piece of design is used that would make any engineer proud. The veins that drain these superficial tissues are linked up with the deep veins through a number of perforations in the fibrous sheath. Each linking or communication vein is guarded by a one-way valve. As we walk, the muscle pump squeezes the deep veins in our legs; blood is pushed upwards towards the heart; and the negative pressure within the deep veins sucks in blood through the communicating veins from the skin and the fat. As we shall see in the following chapter, it is when this brilliant but delicate piece of apparatus is unable to do its job for some reason that varicose veins develop.

Which veins become varicose?

The superficial, or surface veins of our legs, and these are the ones that develop into varicose veins, are called long and short saphenous veins. The word saphenous comes from the Arabic word meaning 'casily visible' and certainly the lower-most part of the veins of the leg, around the ankle and on the front of the foot, are visible in perfectly normal people. The long saphenous vein can be seen just in front of your ankle joint on its inner side. The vein runs upwards along the inner side of your leg, behind the kneecap into the thigh. It then passes through the fibrous sheath of your leg at the groin to enter the femoral (thigh) vein. This is the most important of the many linking veins between the surface and deep veins of the leg and it is here that the surgeon often has to operate in those patients with severe varicose veins (see page 50).

The short saphenous vein begins behind the outer side of your ankle and runs up behind the leg to the back of your knee. Here it too penetrates through the fibrous sheath of your leg to enter a large deep vein called the popliteal, which changes its name into the femoral a little higher in the thigh. As well as these two major linking veins, at the groin and behind the knee, there are many other connections between the surface and deep veins, and each is guarded by

The surface and deep vein systems of the leg

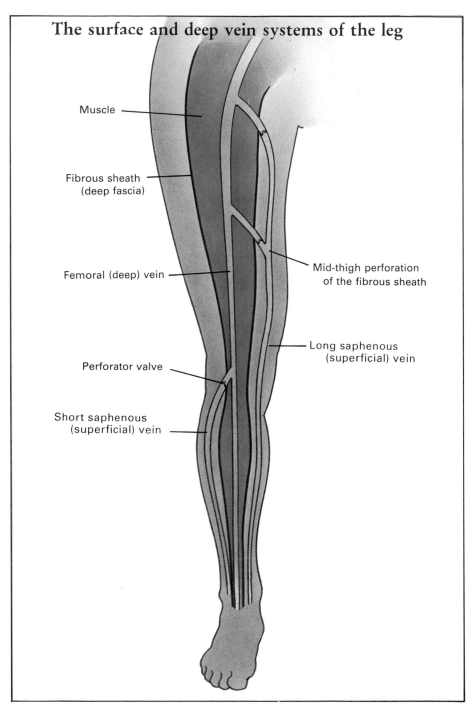

Muscle

Fibrous sheath
(deep fascia)

Femoral (deep) vein

Perforator valve

Short saphenous
(superficial) vein

Mid-thigh perforation
of the fibrous sheath

Long saphenous
(superficial) vein

A diagram to show the surface and deep veins of the leg. There are two main surface veins, both connecting with the deep veins through the muscle sheath.

a valve that allows blood to flow only from the surface to the deep veins – when everything is working normally, that is.

The fine structure of veins

If you look at a leg vein under a microscope (see photograph below), you will see that it is made up of three layers. The innermost layer is a smooth, shining membrane made up of flattened cells with irregular outlines that fit together rather like a jigsaw puzzle. The middle layer contains the elastic tissue that allows the vein to stretch, and there are also some muscle fibres that allow the vein to contract. The outermost layer is really just a coat of a connective tissue.

The surface veins have quite a considerable amount of smooth muscle in their walls, far more than in the deep veins. This means that the surface veins can contract in response to injury or cold and may expand in response to heat and to chemicals, such as the female sex hormones. The deep veins, on the other hand, are much more like passive tubes which are emptied by the squeezing effect of surrounding muscles when these contract, and by the force of gravity

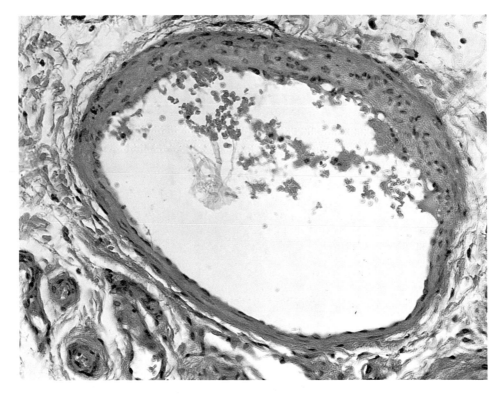

A cross-section of a vein under the microscope.

when you keep your leg raised.

The valves in the leg veins, whose function, as we have seen, is to help the blood flow back towards the heart, consist of a double fold of the smooth innermost layer of the vein with the addition of a certain amount of smooth muscle and connective tissue from the middle and outer layers. It is a failure of these valves that is the basic cause of varicose veins in our legs. If the defective valve is in one of the veins joining the surface and deep vein systems, the part of the surface vein normally protected by this valve is suddenly made to cope with a high-pressure back-flow of blood from the muscle pump of the leg. The vein's walls expand to cope with the influx of extra blood. In turn, this piece of dilated vein puts pressure on neighbouring valves because, as the vein swells, the valve edges can no longer reach each other in the closed position. So, gradually, often in a time scale measured in years, valve after valve becomes unable to operate and expansion, or dilation, of the surface vein system becomes widespread. If the first valve to break down is at the back of your knee, where the short saphenous vein ends, then the veins

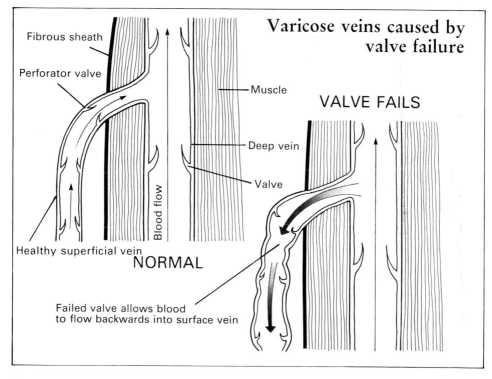

If a valve between the surface and deep leg veins fails, the back flow of blood swells the surface vein, which becomes varicose.

at the back of the calf are affected. If it is the valve in your goin, at the end of the long saphenous vein, then dilations may occur down the inner side of your thigh and the inner side of the calf. There could be other dilations because of the failure of any of the other linking veins scattered throughout the leg.

It seems incredible that so much worry, embarrassment, pain and misery can and does depend on the proper working of these tiny flaps of tissue within the veins of our legs. In the next chapter I shall be looking at the likely reasons why they go wrong.

3 WHAT CAUSES VARICOSE VEINS?

Now why should a valve become ineffective? There are, we believe, quite a number of causes, although I must say here that doctors are hampered by a lack of real research into the early stages of varicose veins. After all, we cannot reproduce varicose veins experimentally in animals to study this condition in the laboratory, and no one is particularly anxious for us to remove his or her early varicose veins and put them under a microscope so that we can investigate the earliest changes that take place in this process.

Failure of valves in the young

First, although we do not know for sure, we believe that the varicose veins beginning in young adults may be due to a very early defect of one or more of the valves. Perhaps the valves actually fail to develop, and there is some evidence that people with varicose veins have fewer valves along the course of the major superficial veins than is normal. It may be that in some people there is a fault in the development of the muscle and elastic tissue in the valve walls.

The protective valves may have developed normally but then have become damaged subsequently. This could be due, for example, to a thrombosis, or clotting, which eventually disappears but leaves behind a damaged valve. Or it may follow an injury to the leg, perhaps completely forgotten about, but enough to produce the defect.

Thrombosis and varicose veins

Sometimes varicose veins appear after a severe thrombosis involving the deep veins that drain the muscles of the calf or the thigh. The thrombosis may occur after a major operation, a serious accident or childbirth. The thrombosed deep vein is first completely blocked with a blood clot but, although this quite rapidly clears, the delicate valves may be permanently damaged as a result. Damage to the valves in the deep veins prevents the leg muscles from pumping blood out efficiently so that there is a build up of high pressure in these veins which is then transmitted to the linking veins and back into the superficial veins. These in their turn become swollen and varicose. (See diagram on page 24.)

Once the valve system has been damaged, a number of other factors may encourage the formation of varicose veins. These include prolonged standing, pregnancy and possibly the climate.

When you're on your feet all day

If you are one of those people in an occupation that keeps them on their feet a great deal you will have no trouble from your superficial veins provided the valves are perfectly healthy. But if these are defective in any way, the high pressure that arises in veins when you're in the standing position will undoubtedly increase your chances of developing varicose veins.

Pregnancy

This has long been known to have an effect on varicose veins. Many women complain that their varicose veins become more prominent and uncomfortable during pregnancy and many even claim that they originated during pregnancy. There are two reasons for this. The

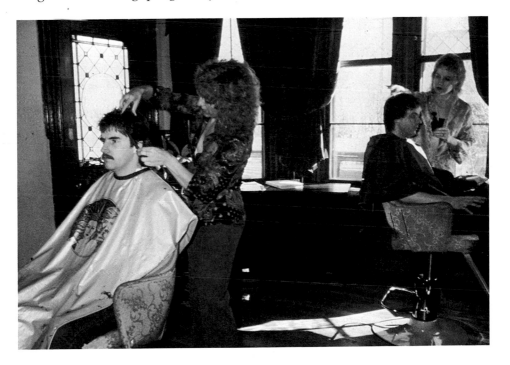

Contrary to popular belief, being on your feet all day does not actually cause varicose veins. Although if you have them already it may make them worse in the long run.

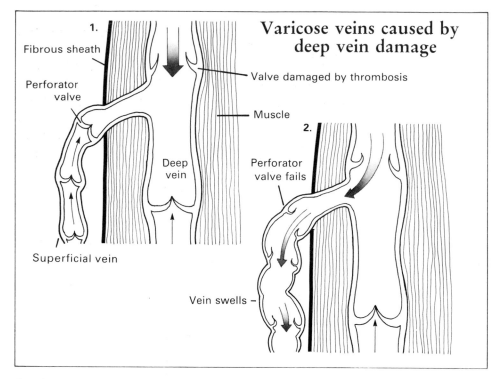

A valve damaged by thrombosis in a deep vein allows blood to flow backwards and distend the surface veins.

first is that the enlarged womb presses on the veins within the mother's pelvis and this slows the return of blood from the legs to the heart. This means that pressure builds up within these veins and is transmitted all the way back to the superficial veins of the leg which then expand. Second, we know that female sex hormones (oestrogens) relax the muscles in the veins and this also increases the tendency of the veins to expand. Interestingly, the uncomfortable varicose veins of pregnancy rapidly improve once the baby has been born and these two aggravating factors have been removed.

Varicose veins in pregnancy is such an important topic that I shall be examining the problem more fully in chapter four.

Heat
A warm environment or climate can also result in the swelling of the surface veins of the leg and people with varicose veins who live or work under such conditions will certainly notice that their varicose veins become rather more swollen and uncomfortable.

Garters

I am often asked if tight, constricting articles of clothing around the legs can produce varicose veins. There doesn't seem to be any evidence that this is so. However, it is true that if you already have varicose veins the tight constriction around the leg made by a garter, say, will produce stagnation of the blood in the dilated veins below the constriction, and this may well lead to clotting of the blood and an attack of thrombosis in the leg. Long, tight boots, which become fashionable every now and then, compress the leg along its length and are probably entirely harmless even if you have varicose veins. Most people today wear sensible, non-constricting comfortable clothes. Those who do wear garters, suspenders and so on, need not worry that they will *cause* varicose veins. They should be avoided, however, if varicose veins are already there. So too should any other cause of stagnation of the blood such as prolonged sitting or standing still.

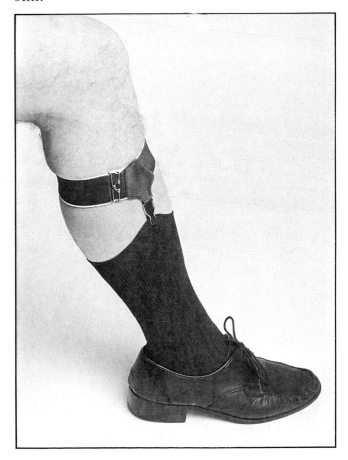

Wearing tight garters certainly won't give you varicose veins. But if you do suffer from them, garters may lead to an attack of clotting in the leg.

Is there a common factor?

Now that we have a fair idea of what varicose veins are and what causes them, the question that inevitably arises is why do they seem to be so common? You only have to keep your eyes open at the seaside or at a swimming pool to realize just how common they are. Yet, as far as I know, varicose veins occur only in human beings and although I have looked carefully at many animals, both in their natural surroundings and in zoos, I have never seen a single example of varicose veins in any other species. No doubt this is the result of the upright position unique to humans, so that the veins lying in the superficial tissues of our legs come to lie 3–4 ft (90–120 cm) below the heart, unsupported except for a little surrounding fibrous and fatty tissue. But if that were the case then practically the whole human race would be afflicted, whereas we know this is not so.

There are four important factors that many doctors believe have some bearing on the frequency of varicose veins – heredity, race, diet and your sex.

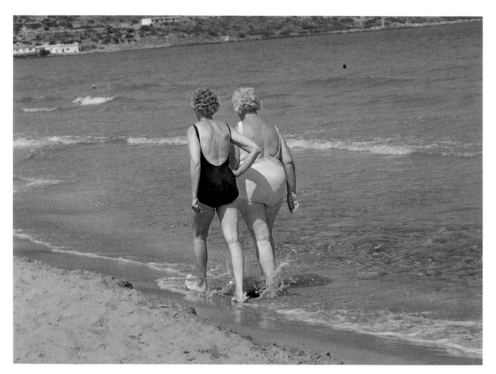

Around 20 per cent of the Western population will have varicose veins at some time in their lives. And nowhere is this more evident than on the beach in summer.

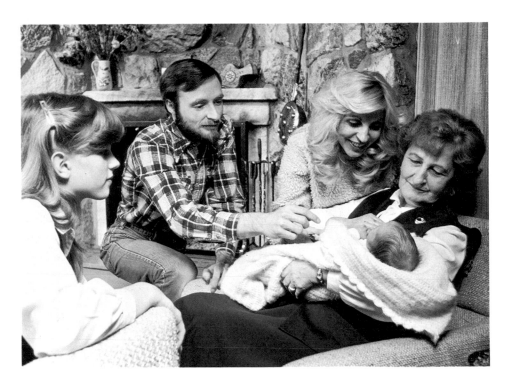

All the evidence points to varicose veins being hereditary. Three out of four sufferers have close family with the same condition.

Heredity

There seems to be quite a lot of evidence to support the idea that varicose veins are inherited. If this is true, then some good advice to any young person wishing to avoid them is to be very careful in the choice of his or her parents! In fact something like three-quarters of all patients with varicose veins have other close members of the family who have the same condition. This may be one or both parents, one or more brothers and sisters, and often other close relatives – uncles, aunts, cousins or grandparents. When varicose veins start in the early teens (and every now and then we see varicose veins beginning in school children) almost invariably there is a clear family history of this condition. In one study of patients with varicose ulcers, no fewer than nine out of ten were able to recall close relatives who suffered from varicose veins.

Race

From the racial point of view (and this again may represent an inherited factor) it is well known that peoples of the more technologically advanced nations of Europe, North America and Australasia are particularly prone to varicose veins. Indeed, it has been estimated that between 10 and 20 per cent of the white population of the Western world suffers from varicose veins to some extent. Although varicose veins do occur among peoples in Africa, on the Indian subcontinent and in the Far East, they are certainly far less common than in the Western world. Some experts have even gone so far as to say that varicose veins are not found in Africans. I can certainly vouch, from my own observations, that this is not so, and I have seen some examples of very bad varicose veins in people marching through parts of the East African bush.

It is true that surgeons working in the Third World report that they rarely have to operate on this condition, but we have to be very careful about using hospital statistics to back up arguments about racial differences in the occurrence of varicose veins. It is reasonable to assume that most Africans or Indians will be more concerned about the basic problems of life such as getting enough to eat, than with the cosmetic appearance of their legs. However, even taking this into consideration, population surveys have confirmed that there are marked racial variations.

Interestingly enough, varicose veins are frequently found in the black population of the United States. It is a fact that raises fascinating arguments as to whether their occurrence can be explained by intermarriage – today only a minority of black Americans are of pure African ancestry – or whether other factors such as diet and exercise have some part to play.

Do varicose veins result from our Western lifestyle?

Let us look a little more closely at some of the differences between so-called civilized Westerners and people living in, say, rural communities in the Third World. Is the widespread occurrence of varicose veins among Westerners compared with their relative absence among Third World peoples due entirely to heredity or can some other factors be at work?

Anyone who has travelled at all extensively will immediately realize that the two most significant differences between these two groups of people are their very different diets and their very different levels of physical activity.

Diet Primitive man existed on a diet of fruit, vegetables and unprocessed grains with the occasional luxury of meat, if he was lucky. This situation hasn't changed much today throughout most of the

Third World. In order to take in an adequate amount of energy, large amounts of these foodstuffs must be consumed daily and, in consequence, the rural communities in much of Africa, the Indian subcontinent and the Far East, for example, have plenty of bulk, or roughage, in their diet, most of it in the form of cereal, fruit and vegetable fibre, which is the substance that forms the cell wall of the plant and provides its rigid structure. As a consequence, they pass large, soft, bulky stools, with a rapid transit time through the intestine.

Contrast this situation with ours – their sophisticated Western cousins – who have a diet of highly refined foods. Bread in the Western world is processed so that much of the coarse fibre of the grain is removed. Instead of chewing on a sugar cane, with its high fibre content, we get pure refined sugar out of a packet. The low bulk of our refined food is reflected in the much smaller amount of stool that we pass daily, often in the form of constipated pellets. Indeed, studies comparing the amount of bowel action passed daily by the average English town-dweller and the average African farmer show figures of $3 \cdot 5$ oz (100 g) as compared to $17 \cdot 5$ oz (500 g).

Human beings have been used to the high-roughage diet for millions of years. Only in the last one hundred years or so has the highly refined diet that we are now used to been introduced to certain communities – those of Western Europe, North America, Australasia and the white population of Southern Africa. We should not be surprised to learn that in such a short time our large intestines have not been able to adapt to the change. The consequence is the constipation that is such a common complaint in civilized communities. There is also good evidence to show that diverticular disease, in which small blown-out pouches develop in the wall of the colon (the end of the large intestine) is associated with this diet and that the symptoms due to both constipation and diverticular disease can be controlled, in the majority of cases, simply by introducing adequate amounts of dietary fibre into our diet. Dr Denis Burkitt has produced an excellent book in this series, *Don't Forget Fibre in Your Diet* (called *Eat Right to Stay Healthy and Enjoy Life More* in the United States) which I can certainly recommend you to read on this subject.

While completely agreeing that many of the bowel problems I have to deal with in my practice are due to our peculiar dietary habits, I personally would like to see more evidence to connect the Western refined diet with the varicose veins. Nevertheless, there are many people who attach considerable weight to the reasoning and certainly we should not discount anything that may increase our knowledge about varicose veins and through it, our ability to apply methods of treatment and prevention.

Those experts who think that our low-fibre diets have a direct bearing on the high percentage of varicose veins in the West argue along these lines: Animals who walk on all fours have a large intestine that hangs down against the abdominal wall (a glance at the bulging belly of a horse, dog or cat will confirm this). In man, in his upright position, the lower part of the large bowel sinks down into the pelvis. If the bowel is loaded with constipated stool it compresses the large veins (iliac veins) in the pelvis, which in turn drain the veins of the leg. To make matters worse, the straining needed to evacuate your bowel when you have constipation will produce an increase in the pressure on the veins in the abdominal cavity and this too will be transmitted to the veins of the leg. The increased pressure build-up in the leg veins, over the years, will lead to deterioration of the valves and hence to varicose veins. Dr Burkitt and others have pointed out yet a third possibility. Primitive man empties his bowel in the squatting position. This position prevents pressure being transmitted down the leg veins, but this is not the case in the comfortably seated position adopted by lavatory-trained Western races.

Exercise   Another important and obvious difference between our two populations, the sophisticated and the more primitive, is in the amount of walking and exercise we undertake. Here in the West we spend much of our time standing still at the work-bench, sitting at our desks or in front of our television sets; African or Indian peasants, on the other hand, spend much of their time walking about. Now, while they are walking about, the muscle pumps of their legs work hard to return blood in the veins to the heart. While we are sitting down or standing still we have a stagnant column of high-pressure blood in our leg veins. This, enthusiasts argue, must be an important factor in pointing to the origin of varicose veins.

One argument against the theory that modern ways of life are at the root of varicose veins is the simple fact that this problem is so much more common in women than in men. Yet both men and women get just as constipated as each other and both spend about the same amount of time standing or sitting. So, if the diet and exercise factors are to be of overwhelming importance, then there should be very little difference in the number of varicose vein cases between the sexes.

Even if we could prove that our modern way of life has something to do with the cause of varicose veins, what can we do about preventing the development of varicose veins in future generations? It is difficult enough to convince people that they should give up smoking, even with all the overwhelming evidence of its strong association with cancer, heart disease and chronic bronchitis (though not, incidentally, with varicose veins). Can people ever be persuaded to give up the refined carbohydrate and over-processed foods and return to a more natural diet of at least adequate fibre content, or to give up the car and the television and walk ten miles a day in order possibly to prevent the development of varicose veins? Although it seems highly unlikely, it is a goal towards which everyone wishing to live a healthier, happier life can aspire even if we can't, for the moment, prove conclusively that it will even prevent our varicose veins. There is no doubt, however, that once you have varicose veins, diet and exercise should play an important rôle in their treatment; and there are recommendations on both in chapters six and seven.

Your sex

Any doctor will tell you that he sees three or four times as many women as men suffering from varicose veins. One obvious reason for this is that women are more likely to report for treatment for cosmetic reasons. Few women would remain unperturbed by their unsightly black and blue knotted veins when wearing a dress or swimwear. Another reason why fewer men report this condition to their doctor is the hairiness of male legs. It is not uncommon for a man to have his legs shaved in hospital for some surgical procedure – a cartilage operation, for example – and to discover, for the first time, that he has a considerable crop of unsuspected varicose veins hidden beneath the hair.

Even so, this certainly does not account for the fact that the number of women with varicose veins far outweighs the number of men. This is confirmed by population surveys and also by the fact that haemorrhage, phlebitis and ulceration, complications that bring practically all sufferers to hospital, are much more often seen in women than in men. It may well be that, as we said earlier, this tendency for women to be more susceptible to varicose veins has something to do with the female sex hormones, oestrogens, acting on the muscle in the walls of the veins and relaxing them. I shall be dealing with this more fully in the next chapter.

4 THE PILL, PREGNANCY AND VARICOSE VEINS

The contraceptive pill

It is estimated that more than 3 million women in Britain are taking one or other of the hormone-based contraceptive pills available today and that this has become the most popular form of contraception throughout the Western world. As we shall see later on in the chapter, there is a well-recognized relationship between pregnancy and varicose veins. It seems sensible, therefore, to look for any possible link between the pill and varicose veins. There are two questions to be answered: First, does the pill produce varicose veins? and second, are there any dangers for a woman on the pill who is already suffering from varicose veins?

Before we can answer these questions, we had better spend a few moments finding out what the various pills actually do. The clue to how hormones can be used as contraceptive agents was found when people realized that during pregnancy the mother does not get pregnant again! This is because the hormones produced by the placenta, or after-birth, during pregnancy – oestrogens and progesterone – prevent further eggs (or ova) being set free by the ovary until the pregnancy has ended.

When about fifty years ago oestrogens were being used in the treatment of painful periods, doctors found that they also prevented the release of eggs from the ovary. Ten years later it was found that various laboratory-produced progesterone-like chemicals had a similar effect on the ovary. In 1956 the first big trial was carried out in Puerto Rico using Enavid, a progesterone agent. This was soon followed by the modern contraceptive pills, the great majority of which are made up of a mixture of oestrogen and a progestagen – a progesterone-type hormone.

Side-effects
About twenty years ago evidence started to accumulate showing that there was a very small increase in the risk of thrombosis, or clotting of the blood vessels, in women taking the pill. Cases of coronary

thrombosis (heart attacks), cerebral thrombosis (strokes) and thrombosis of the deep veins of the leg were reported as well as, in very rare cases, clotting within the arteries supplying blood to the intestine. I must stress here that the risk of all these is actually very small. For example, in 1974 a report was published in Britain on 23,000 women who were taking contraceptive pills compared with another 23,000 who were not. The results suggested that the risk of clotting was something like six times greater in women on the pill compared with those who were not. But I emphasize that the numbers are small. In another study, the statistics show that out of every 200,000 women taking the pill, 3 might be expected to die of some clotting illness each year in those under the age of thirty-five. The risk was rather greater, just less than 8 per 200,000, in women over the age of thirty-five. To put this danger into perspective, one authority said that when a father buys a motorboat he introduces a tenfold greater risk of sudden death in his family than could be associated with his wife taking the pill! Against this we must also place, of course, all the risks and dangers that are associated with unwanted pregnancies.

Since these statistics have become available, the amount of oestrogen in the two-hormone pill has been reduced by 50 per cent, so it may be that the possible dangers of the contraceptive pill have been reduced to an even lower level, though it will probably be some time before we know this for sure. There are pills containing only progestagen but there is still a problem of balance – finding a dose small enough not to produce irregular periods, and also large enough to make sure of contraception. Statistics for the progestagen-only pills give a rate of 2 to 3 pregnancies for every 100 woman years, compared with less than 0.5 with the two-hormone pill.

Armed with this information about the chemical make-up of the pill, and its effect on the blood, we can now look at the pill's effect on varicose veins.

The pill and varicose veins
First, although we know that oestrogen relaxes veins and is partly responsible for the expansion of veins in the leg that occurs during pregnancy, we can find no definite evidence that varicose veins have become more widespread since the introduction of contraceptive pills. There is no reason, therefore, why you should not take the pill because of fear that varicose veins may develop as a result.

If you already have varicose veins, however, particularly if these are extensive, or if you have had an attack of phlebitis, or clotting (see page 82) in the veins, your doctor is unlikely to prescribe the contraceptive pill containing oestrogen, more especially if you are over the age of thirty-five or forty, because we know that the risk of thrombosis in that age range becomes greater. It would be better to use some other form of contraception, or your gynaecologist might prescribe a pill containing only progestagen. The very slight risk in using the pill is also probably further reduced if you have had your varicose veins cleared up completely either by surgery or by injection treatment (see pages 41–52).

There is one very important practical point. Some women have reported that their calf muscles ache and they associate this with being on the pill. Naturally both they and their doctors will be anxious about the possibility of this being a sign that their varicose veins or deep veins are clotting. Medical examination can speedily decide whether the aching calf muscles are due simply to cramps in the muscle or to varicose veins. If cramps are diagnosed, changing the pill to one of a lower oestrogen content sometimes relieves the symptoms but, if not, it may be necessary to change to some other method of contraception.

Because of a slight increase in the risk of thrombosis in veins when you're on the pill, many surgeons advise their patients to stop using this form of contraception for four to six weeks before an operation – and this includes, of course, having surgery for your varicose veins. You can start taking the pill again two weeks after surgery.

Varicose veins in pregnancy

One of the problems that shows early in many pregnancies is the appearance of varicose veins or, if the woman already has them, then she notices that they are suddenly getting much worse.

The veins show up as one or more of the following:

1. Straightforward varicosities of the surface veins of the leg.
2. Development of broken veins (spider naevi) in the skin of the thighs.
3. Vulval varicosities.

There are two reasons for the development of new varicose veins or the worsening of those already existing in your leg during the early months of pregnancy. First, there is the presence of the enlarging uterus (womb), which presses on the pelvic veins and obstructs the drainage of blood from your legs. The rise in pressure behind the obstruction will be transmitted, of course, downwards into the surface veins of your legs. The second reason is the rise in the level of sex hormones in your blood. These hormones relax the muscle tissue in the vein walls and so increase the likelihood of their swelling.

Hormones and your veins

There seems little doubt that the effect of hormones on the veins is an important one and may well be the reason why varicose veins are several times more common in women than in men. Hormones may also be responsible for a commonly observed phenomenon in women with varicose veins – they tend to find that their veins are worse and more uncomfortable just before a menstrual period.

Because the hormonal effect occurs quite early in pregnancy, the sudden development of varicose veins – or their becoming painful – is looked upon as being almost as significant as a missed period in

One cause of varicose veins during pregnancy is the womb pressing on the pelvic veins, thus transmitting pressure back down to the leg veins.

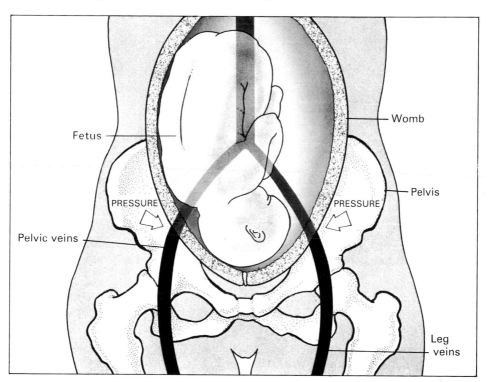

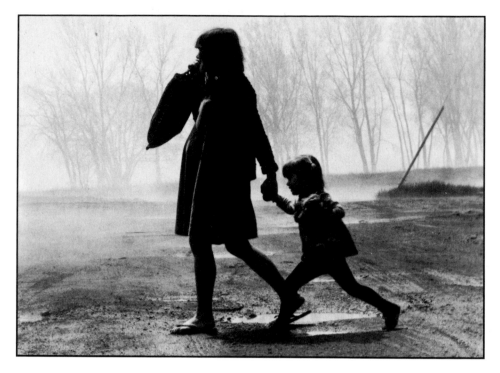

For the mother-to-be, a good long walk every day is of tremendous value, not only in helping to control her varicose veins, but also for her general health and well-being.

making an early diagnosis of pregnancy!

After the arrival of your baby, the varicose veins that appeared during pregnancy may disappear completely, and even established varicose veins will certainly become much improved. However, it is also true to say that the varicose veins are very likely to reappear again at the next pregnancy and become more marked in further pregnancies.

Treatment

A great many doctors, especially in Britain, are very much against the treatment of varicose veins during pregnancy. In the first place, we can almost guarantee that your legs will improve, even go back to normal, after your baby is born. In the second place, doctors are very cautious indeed about submitting pregnant women to any sort of therapy, when it involves either an operation or injections, which they do not consider absolutely essential either to the health of the mother or the well-being of the expected child. It is virtually impossible for a minor operation or an injection of a varicose vein to affect your baby in any way. My old friend Professor George Fegan of Dublin has told me in the course of many conversations how he has personally dealt with large numbers of pregnant women by injection treatment with complete safety to both mother and child. Nevertheless, if after treatment for a vein there should be any blemish at all in the baby, then it would take a very strong-minded parent indeed not to think that *perhaps* wanting to get rid of ugly or uncomfortable veins might have harmed the child. When that happens, even the strongest reassurances cannot entirely help.

Support stockings and exercise   The standard treatment of varicose veins in pregnancy is therefore to fit the mother with full-length, properly fitting elastic support stockings. Put the stockings on first thing in the morning, on getting up, wear them throughout the day and leave them off only at night. Cosmetically the modern stockings have an acceptable appearance if ordinary nylon stockings are worn over them. Exercise is excellent; a good brisk walk helps to pump the blood out of the leg veins and 3 miles (5 km) a day is a reasonable target. Avoid garters or undergarments that are too tight, as they only aggravate the congestion of blood in leg veins. See chapter seven for more detailed advice on exercise and elastic stockings.

Put your feet up!   You will soon learn the great value of putting your legs up during the day whenever possible and also sleeping either with your heels raised on pillows while in bed at night or else with the foot of the bed raised about 12 in (30 cm) above the head by means of a strong box, bricks, or some other firm support.

Once pregnancy is over, both you and your doctor can assess whether or not the varicose veins, now much improved, are going to need treatment. If they are not severe, there is much to be said for putting off treatment until you have given birth to your last child, but if the veins are causing any discomfort, then any time from a few weeks after delivery is perfectly satisfactory for either injection or surgical treatment, whichever of the two is right for your particular condition.

Spider naevi
These tiny dilated blood vessels in the skin of the thighs often seem to make their first appearance during pregnancy, but they cause no harm and should be left strictly alone. I shall be dealing with these in more detail on page 93.

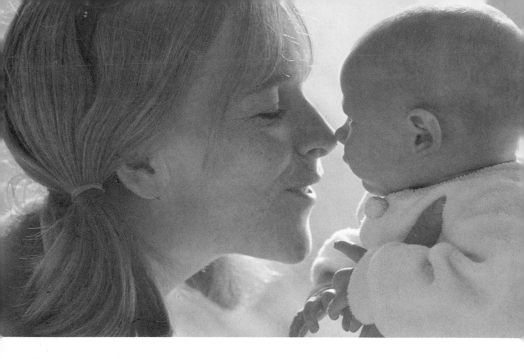

If you have severe varicose veins, you can have them treated by injections or surgery from a few weeks after your baby is born.

Vulval veins

It is during pregnancy that the surface veins of the vulva (around the entrance to the vagina) and on the inner side of the top of the thigh sometimes expand and become varicose. Indeed, they have been known to develop quite rapidly and can be a rather alarming sight by about the third or fourth month of the pregnancy.

Although ugly, and indeed sometimes rather frightening in appearance, these veins very rarely give rise to any trouble such as bleeding or clotting either during the pregnancy or during delivery. As soon as the baby is born, they begin to shrink and often disappear completely.

No treatment is advised during pregnancy but you can be assured that the condition is completely harmless and will greatly improve once your baby has been delivered. It is true that the veins may still be visible after your confinement and may require surgical removal through one or two tiny skin incisions. Although some doctors recommend injection treatment for these vulval varicose veins, most surgeons consider that a small operation is more effective and less uncomfortable. The whole question of treatment of varicose veins is an important one, of course, and in the next chapter I shall be considering the pros and cons of the different methods.

5 TREATMENT

When you consult your doctor about varicose veins, he will offer you one of four courses of treatment: 1. Do nothing at all. 2. Wear elastic stockings. 3. Have injection treatment. 4. Have surgery.

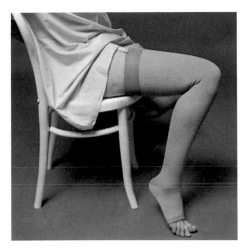
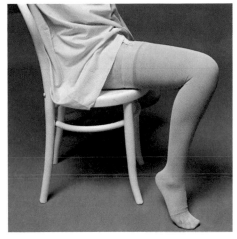

A long elastic support stocking . . . covered by an ordinary stocking to improve its appearance.

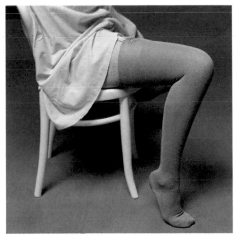

A cosmetic support stocking.

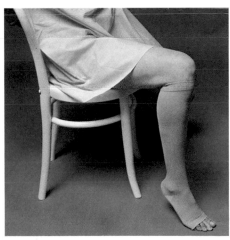

A short support stocking.

No treatment

If you have only very mild varicose veins which are giving little if any trouble, your doctor will usually advise you to leave well alone. Varicose veins do not suddenly become much worse, and minor degrees of swollen veins are not subject to the various complications I have set out in chapter eight. Often a doctor finds that there is some underlying anxiety behind a patient's request for treatment. This may be because a relative, very often the mother, has been plagued with all the burdens of a bad leg (probably a varicose ulcer) for many years. It is, I suppose, perfectly reasonable for her offspring, discovering the first trace of a varicose vein, to imagine that he or she, too, is rapidly going to develop severe ulceration.

Perhaps you are one of those young women who have chubby legs or thick ankles and who hope that treatment of one or two tiny veins in the leg might improve your appearance. I want to say here that any therapy for your varicose veins is only going to produce disappointment, as a look at chapter six will tell you.

You may belong to a third category of patients who either do not suffer from varicose veins at all or whose minor varicose veins simply disguise other causes of aching and discomfort in the legs (again, see chapter eight). Here, obviously, your doctor will need to find out the real cause of the symptoms and use appropriate treatment.

Now, if your veins are cosmetically unpleasant or are producing symptoms of discomfort, or if there have been any of the complications which sometimes accompany varicose veins (see pages 82–93), then the time has come to decide on active treatment. The aim of all forms of treatment is to keep the affected veins empty of blood.

Elastic stockings

The veins in your legs can be supported and compressed by elastic stockings, but these will not by themselves cure varicose veins. The stockings are, however, extremely useful in a number of categories. They are very helpful to elderly patients whose general health is not good enough for even the safe and fairly minor treatments that we use to cure varicose veins. The stockings are also useful in giving temporary relief to very overweight patients while they slim themselves down in preparation for more specific treatment. As we saw in chapter four, support stockings are also valuable for varicose veins during pregnancy.

A whole range of elastic stockings is now available for varicose vein sufferers. You will find that cosmetically they are quite acceptable, and indeed ordinary stockings can be worn over them to improve their appearance still further. It is important to remember that, with repeated washing, elastic stockings lose their elasticity and when this happens you will need new ones.

What do elastic stockings do?

Their action is simply to compress the swollen veins on the surface of your leg, emptying them into the deep vein system where the muscle pump can return the blood to the heart. To get the maximum benefit from the stockings remember two simple rules:

1. Once the leg is well supported, you should walk about as much as possible. The elastic stocking gently but firmly presses the swollen surface veins and squeezes the blood in them back into the deep muscle pump. The action of the muscles is to return the blood to the heart and this, of course, is tremendously increased by exercise. A good 3-mile (5-km) walk each day will work wonders!

2. Keep the leg raised when you are not walking and the muscle pump is not in use. Take off the stockings at night; there is no need to wear them in bed. Once in bed, however, the veins should be kept empty by sleeping with your heel raised above your knee and your knee above your hip. This can be achieved either with one or two pillows placed under your legs or else by getting the foot of the bed raised up on a strong box, some bricks or any other technique that you or your family can devise. I will give some more advice about wearing elastic stockings in chapter seven.

Injection treatment

The injection treatment of varicose veins is well over a century old. A solution of iron chloride was the first substance to be used to produce the seemingly paradoxical healing processes of clotting and inflammation in the veins. This was followed by a weak solution of phenol, then sodium salicylate and then a mixture of quinine and urethane. Although successes were achieved, the body's reaction to

Injection treatment

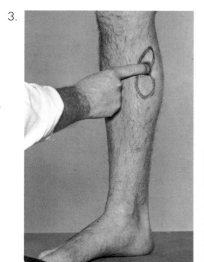

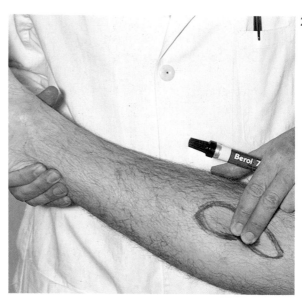

1. The varicose veins are marked out on the leg.   2. With the leg elevated, the failed perforator valve is located.

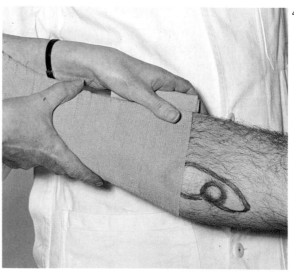

3. The patient stands and the surgeon presses on the perforator valve to confirm that this now controls the varicose vein.   4. The leg is bandaged from the toes to just below the site of the injection.

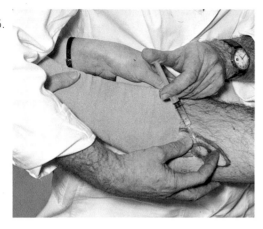

5. The perforator valve is injected using a very fine needle – this should be almost painless!

6. A pad is placed over the injection site.

7. The bandage is continued up to the knee.

8. Finally, the leg is supported by an elastic stocking over the bandage.

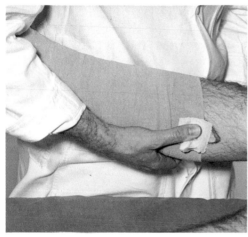

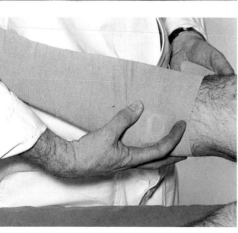

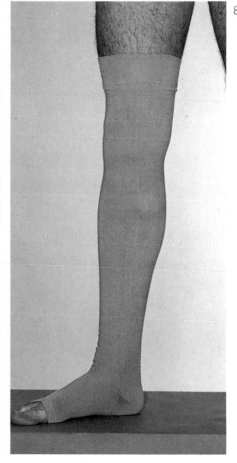

these substances was occasionally severe and the long-term results were not particularly good.

How does it work?
Much credit goes to Professor George Fegan of Dublin for the injection therapy we use today. As a young surgeon, in 1950 he was put in charge of the varicose vein clinic at the famous Dublin maternity hospital, the Rotunda. He found himself faced with some thirty new patients each week but with no hospital beds for operative treatment. He therefore resolved to refine what had, until then, been a rather hit-and-miss injection method and the technique he devised forms the basis of the treatment given in most varicose vein clinics throughout the world today.

Professor Fegan's method is based on good physiological and anatomical principles. First the surgeon has to find the points along your leg where the varicose veins penetrate through the sheath of fibrous tissue that surrounds the leg muscles and drain into the deep veins. These penetrating, or communicating veins are called the perforators (often nicknamed the 'blow-outs').

In order to find the sites of the perforating veins, the surgeon will make you stand up and then mark with a pen the general distribution of the varicose veins on your leg. He will then ask you to lie down on the examination couch and your leg will be raised to empty the veins. The surgeon will then carefully feel along the leg to find the little defects that mark the spots where the surface veins penetrate through the fibrous sheath of the leg into the deep veins. These points often correspond to particularly large bulges in the varicose veins themselves.

The surgeon will then use his pen to mark these points on the skin. He next presses each of these perforators with his fingers and you will then be asked to stand up again. It is at this point that the surgeon discovers if his search has been successful, for it will be obvious in the standing position that the veins are controlled at these points of pressure. When he takes his finger off one of these points, the varicose vein being fed from this point will then be seen to fill with blood and to swell. If the vein fills before he has taken his finger off then he realizes that he has missed a perforator and repeats the test until all the blow-outs are localized and marked.

An injection of an irritant solution will be given into these sites which will set up an intense but controlled inflammation. The idea is that the body's defence and healing mechanism will immediately start to close off the blow-out by the creation of scar tissue, thus

44

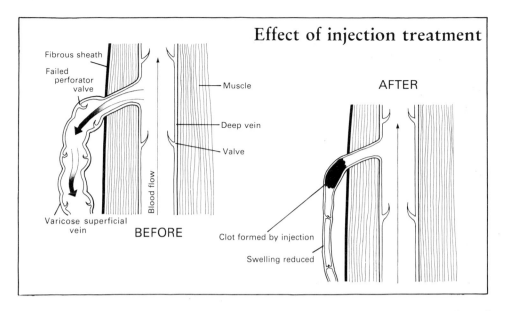

Fibrous sheath
Failed perforator valve
Muscle
AFTER
Deep vein
Valve
Blood flow
Varicose superficial vein
BEFORE
Clot formed by injection
Swelling reduced

The clot formed by the injection closes off the flow of blood into the varicose vein and so reduces the swelling.

stopping the high-pressure back-flow of blood through the varicose vein and reducing the swelling. To make sure that the reaction does not spread to nearby healthy veins, the injection will be given into the vein, which is emptied of blood by raising your leg during the injection. Your leg will then be firmly bandaged from the toes up to above the site of the injection. We used to keep the pressure bandage on for several weeks – which was not at all pleasant for the patient. However, recent experience has shown that this is not necessary. Many surgeons, including myself, recommend keeping the leg bandaged for a week and then using elastic stocking support for another week or two until the leg is quite comfortable. Others have abandoned bandaging completely and tell me their results are just as good. To encourage the flow of blood from the leg and to prevent the slight risk of any extensive clotting of stagnant blood within the veins of the leg, you will be instructed to walk briskly at least 3 miles (5 km) every day, starting with the day of injection. It is also wise to keep your leg raised in bed at night on a couple of pillows.

There are a number of chemical solutions we can use to inject into veins. My own preference is for a substance called sodium tetradecyl sulphate, which is dissolved in an alcoholic solution. The material has, in fact, the properties of a detergent. It probably combines with the protein of the cells lining the wall of the vein, damaging them and causing a brisk local inflammation. It is so highly effective that only a small amount (0·5 to 1 ml) is necessary at any point of injection.

When injection treatment is not possible

Veins that extend up the thigh to the groin are difficult, and in many cases impossible, to compress by bandaging, which many of us regard as an important part of injection therapy. In such cases surgeons usually advise surgical treatment, which I will be describing later on in this chapter.

Very obese patients are almost impossible to treat by injection because it is difficult to find their perforators and even more difficult to bandage their legs satisfactorily so as to keep the veins compressed and empty. Seriously overweight patients are usually put on a vigorous reducing diet. The promise that they will be able to have their veins treated satisfactorily once they have lost weight is usually a great incentive to these sufferers. We will deal with the subject of obesity and losing weight more fully in the next chapter.

Follow-up

Once you have had the injection (or injections) you will be expected to go to your surgeon a week later. The bandages will be removed and the leg examined. At this stage it is usually possible to see if a good result is going to be achieved. It may be, however, that the injection did not create the right amount of inflammation and so will have to be repeated. Sometimes we find that one or more perforators have been missed and these can then be injected at this visit. If you require any further injections, you can be seen again the following week and the process repeated once more. However, once the veins have been successfully injected, I recommend keeping the leg supported during the day with an elastic stocking until the leg is quite comfortable – usually a week or two. The stocking is taken off at night, but the leg should be kept raised in bed on a pillow. Bathing and showering are allowed. At the end of this time, if the treatment has been successful, you will be delighted to find that the treated veins have disappeared completely.

Frequently, where varicose veins affect both legs, patients in a hurry to get the treatment over and done with will ask to have both legs injected at the same time. There is no fixed rule, but on the whole I prefer to get one leg treated completely and then deal with the other after the patient has had a period of freedom. You will find that walking about with both legs bandaged and rather sore is cer-

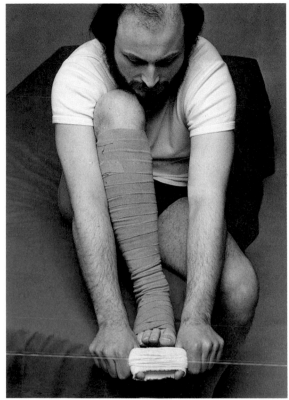

Tubigrip bandaging

Should you need to replace the outer Tubigrip bandage after injection treatment, adopt the following procedure: 1. Roll the bandage together and pull firmly apart between the thumbs. 2. Pull it over the toes, releasing slowly, still keeping it stretched between the thumbs. 3. Continue unrolling until Tubigrip completely covers inner bandage, taking care not to disturb it.

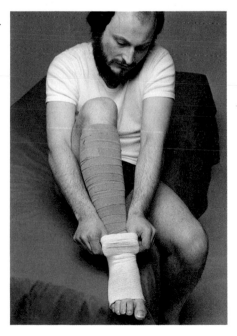

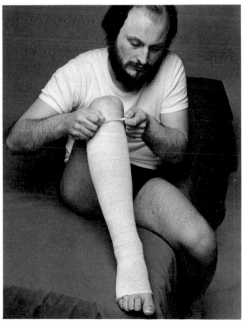

tainly more burdensome than having one good leg. There are always exceptions to any rule, of course, so that if you had some special reason for getting both legs cleared up as quickly as possible – impending marriage for example – or if you can take only a limited time away from full activity, then you may decide to put up with more discomfort for the sake of greater speed.

There is no doubt that having your leg bandaged for a week or more is a nuisance for a number of reasons, not the least of which is the problem of having a bath or shower. A bandaged leg *can* be kept dry either in the tub or under the shower (a shower is the easier of the two) by enclosing it in a large plastic bag and taping the top around the thigh. For this purpose large bags like those used for the disposal of garbage or garden rubbish are ideal. It is also possible to take a shallow bath with the bandaged leg out of the water – but for this you have to be quite athletic!

Is the treatment permanent?
Of course everyone wants to know how successful the treatment will be in the long term. Is it, in fact, permanent? Well, this can not be guaranteed in every case. In some instances the blow-out is not completely obliterated and where this happens a local recurrence of the varicose vein may take place over many months or even years. More likely, though, further varicose veins will develop, either in the same or in the other leg. However, there is no reason why these should not, in turn, be treated quite satisfactorily by injection. You should compare the situation with that of going to the dentist; just because one cavity has been filled does not mean that you will never develop a hole in another tooth nor that the filling itself is going to preserve the tooth for ever.

The great advantage of injection treatment is that the whole thing can be done on an out-patient basis without an anaesthetic and with only very little loss of time from work.

Possible complications
In the majority of patients, injection treatment of varicose veins is a fairly minor procedure. You may experience some pain at the site of the injection for a few days but this can be relieved by mild pain-killers such as aspirin or paracetamol (acetaminophen in the United States). Plenty of walking also helps to keep the leg comfortable and this should be combined with raising the leg whenever you sit or lie down. Avoid standing still. If you find that the inner bandage becomes too tight and uncomfortable, it is worth having it

reapplied at the clinic. If the outer bandage becomes rucked up, dirty or frayed, you can put a new one on yourself (see photographs on page 47). It is a good idea to ask the clinic for some Tubigrip bandage to take home with you for this purpose.

Sometimes, in spite of the greatest care, a little of the injection material will have escaped from the vein into the surrounding tissues. This may produce a dark-coloured area on the skin, which may persist. The patch is quite harmless and is no cause for concern; if you are worried about the appearance of your legs, by all means use a skin-coloured cosmetic cream to camouflage the area. Occasionally the skin in the area where the injection solution has escaped breaks down into a little ulcer. This should slowly heal and simply needs to be covered by a sterile, dry dressing.

Thrombosis (or clotting) of the deep veins of the leg is a rare complication of this form of treatment. With the older injection techniques there is little doubt that some of the solution occasionally passed into the deep veins and damaged them. This is unlikely now with the small amounts of the modern injection solution that we use. On those rare occasions when a thrombosis occurs, it is more likely to be due to the patient not exercising the leg after the injection treatment so that clotting takes place in the sluggish column of blood within the leg muscles. You will avoid this by following the active walking programme that we always advise after injection therapy.

Surgical treatment

This is reserved for patients whose varicose veins are too extensive for injections to be effective. The deciding factor for this is when large varicosities extend up the thigh, often to the groin. These veins are difficult to compress with bandages (particularly if the leg is rather fat) and generally they do not respond at all well to injection treatment. There may, even so, be surgeons who will offer injections under these circumstances, but most would recommend an operation.

Another reason for surgical treatment is that some patients just do not like injections and here an operation to tie off the linking veins lower down the leg might be justifiable. Also, in those cases when patients do not seem to respond to injection treatment an operation may be the only answer.

The operation
If a general anaesthetic is used, this will put you into a deep

sleep until the operation is over. The operation can, if necessary, be carried out under a local anaesthetic, in which case only the area around the vein to be operated on is numbed.

There are two types of operation that can be used to deal with varicose veins. The one most people know about is called the stripping operation. Here the surgeon passes a wire along the length of the varicose vein and uses this to pull out a whole segment of vein. The other operation, which I prefer to use, involves the separation and tying off of the varicose vein.

The operation itself is quite straightforward. As we described in chapter two, the surface vein at the groin – the saphenous vein – enters the deep femoral vein, which lies immediately on the inner side of the main artery of the leg, the femoral artery. The surgeon

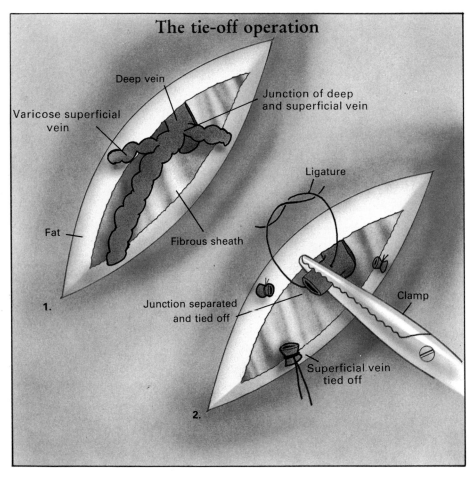

The surgeon will first locate the junction between the deep and superficial veins, and then separate and tie off the two systems.

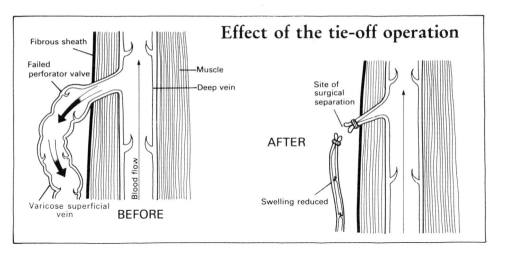

Effect of the tie-off operation

Fibrous sheath

Failed
perforator valve

Muscle

Deep vein

Site of
surgical
separation

AFTER

Blood flow

Varicose superficial
vein

BEFORE

Swelling reduced

By separating the deep veins and the varicose superficial veins, the latter become drained of blood and their swelling is reduced.

makes a short incision over the region of the junction between the long saphenous (surface) vein and the femoral (deep) vein. He divides the little branches of the saphenous vein at the groin and ties them off with fine ligatures of catgut or silk, then he divides and ties off the main trunk of the saphenous vein flush with its point of junction with the femoral vein itself (see diagrams opposite and above). This effectively seals off this main blow-out or incompetent junction between the surface and deep vein systems, thus stopping the high-pressure flow of blood into the varicose surface vein below the junction, and reducing the swelling of the vein. He then closes the small incision in the skin with a few fine stitches (sutures) or skin clips.

In many cases, there are also clumps of unsightly veins lower down the leg. These are carefully marked out with an indelible ink marker before the operation with the patient standing up to render these veins obvious. At operation, a small incision is made over each clump, (often it need only be ¼ to ½ inch in length), and the tortuous dilated vein is dissected free and removed. Sometimes the divided ends of these clumps need to be tied off with fine catgut but often the surgeon relies on compression with a firm dressing and bandage; this reduces the amount of foreign material and subsequent reaction below these little scars.

The patient's rôle

What does the varicose-vein operation involve as far as you the patient are concerned? Many surgeons now carry out varicose vein surgery (under general or local anaesthesia) as a Day Case – admission in the morning, discharge home in the evening. Others prefer an overnight stay, especially if long distances are involved, home care difficult or other social problems make immediate return to your home undesirable. Both legs can safely be dealt with at the same operating session in order to save you a second admission to hospital. After returning home, you can walk about right away and indeed you can often return to light work immediately. The discomfort requires no more than a few pain-relieving pills (such as aspirin or paracetamol/acetaminophen). The stitches and dressings are usually left in for about seven days and are removed when you return to the out-patient clinic.

Wear an elastic stocking – over the bandages at first – when walking about during the day for the next month or so in order to keep the surface veins emptied but you can remove the stocking before retiring to bed, provided that you keep the leg well raised on a couple of pillows during the night.

Pros and cons
Although the operation is quite minor and thousands are performed every year in hospitals in complete safety, I must stress that no operation under the sun is entirely without risk. There may be quite marked bruising beneath the skin or even a small collection of blood (haematoma) which may need to be let out – this is more likely to happen in the case of patients who are overweight. Although rare, a slight infection in the wound may take place because, after all, the groin is not the cleanest part of the body. Again, this is more likely to occur in an overweight patient with rolls of fat at the top of the leg.

It is just possible that you might experience a thrombosis along the course of the surface veins (phlebitis) which may require a few days rest with your leg raised and some mild pain-relieving pills.

So you must weigh up the pros and cons and feel quite sure that the veins are sufficiently irksome – either from their appearance or their discomfort, or both – to warrant the loss of time from work, the inconvenience, the discomfort and even the slight risks of surgical treatment.

Choice of treatment

Doctors are often asked which treatment is better – injections or operation? The answer is that they are not rivals but each has its own applications. Indeed, very often the two methods are combined in dealing with extensive varicose veins.

Injections have an advantage because they can be carried out without your having to come into hospital, also you do not need a general anaesthetic.

Surgery often means a general anaesthetic and a short period of time as an in-patient in hospital. It is the preferred method of treatment in the United States for varicose veins. However, I have already pointed out that in Britain the two methods often have different areas of application: the injections are used for relatively small varicose veins, especially those below the knee, whereas surgery is needed for the large varicose veins extending up to the thigh and groin. The surgeon may have to operate on cases such as this and then use injections to tidy up any further veins lower down the leg.

Recurrence

Varicose veins can be completely cleared up, or certainly greatly improved, by injection or by surgical treatment. However, no doctor would ever claim that the results are permanent. Indeed, something like 20 per cent of people undergoing surgery will develop further varicosities during the five years following treatment. In some cases this is because veins that have been injected have expanded again or a small vein that has not been tied off surgically gradually expands. More often, I believe, these are not recurrences but fresh varicose veins that have developed because of new 'blow-outs'.

This means that a lot of patients are going to be disappointed when they find another varicose vein appearing on the leg. However, on the positive side it must be pointed out that this is quite a slow process so that the leg is not suddenly going to deteriorate into a mass of newly formed varicose veins. It is usually a very simple matter to clear up a newly developed varicosity by means of one or two injections or surgery and this, in turn, will be followed by a good long period of freedom from further trouble.

As I said earlier, if you have a cavity in your tooth filled by the dentist, you are not at all surprised when a few years later a cavity appears in another tooth or that particular filling needs to be changed. I am afraid sufferers from varicose veins must develop the same sort of philosophical approach to their legs.

New valves for old?

You may ask, 'If varicose veins result from damaged valves, why cannot surgeons graft new valves back into the vein, which would restore the mechanism of return of blood to the heart and bring the situation back to normal? After all, surgeons are able to replace heart valves, why not vein valves?

Well, first of all, by the time most patients get to see their surgeon their varicose veins are usually quite pronounced and they have probably progressed to the stage where irreversible expansion and stretching of the veins has occurred. They are by then unlikely to respond to any treatment other than injections or surgery. The second problem is that a reconstructive operation on a vein would be very different from one on an artery and much more likely to be followed by clotting within the vein. The reason is that the flow of blood is much slower and more sluggish in veins than in arteries, and stagnation of blood is a very powerful ally of clotting.

Frankly, for these two reasons, surgeons have been hesitant about trying to devise some way of repairing, replacing or grafting vein valves. Perhaps this will come in the future. I can foresee *preventative* operations for people diagnosed to be at risk from developing varicose veins. These might be youngsters with a very clear family history whose veins are already just starting to expand. Here replacing a faulty valve or two with effective ones might well arrest the development of varicose veins. But that is possibly some time in the future. Meanwhile let us get back to the present and take a look at what happens in the hospital if you should require an operation to treat your veins.

Your stay in hospital

For many patients, coming into hospital for varicose vein surgery is a new, and let's face it, possibly a rather frightening and unpleasant experience. This section scts out to alleviate some of the fears and to give you some idea of what you might expect during your stay.

I must point out that surgeons and hospitals do of course vary from country to country and can also vary widely in their routines from area to area within a country. So do not be too surprised if things prove not to be exactly as stated here.

The fact is that doctors are individualists, and this particularly applies to surgeons. Every experienced surgeon works out the routine that gives the best results in *his* hands, just as any other technician would do. Surgeons therefore differ in the type of stitches they use, how long they keep them in, the brand of skin antiseptic they like to employ, the make of bandage or stocking they utilize, the number of days they recommend you to stay in hospital, and in many other respects. However, your surgeon, his House Surgeon, or the Ward Sister will explain to you which particular routine they employ. They will also inform you about how long you are going to be in hospital, when the stitches or clips are due to be taken out, how long you need to be off work, and so on.

Here is a basic list of the things you should take with you for your short stay in the hospital:

1. Night clothes and a dressing-gown.
2. Slippers.
3. Toilet requisites.
4. A box of soft paper tissues.
5. Plenty of light reading.
6. Writing material and a pen.
7. A bottle of fruit juice or cordial.
8. Some small change – but don't take any valuables if you can possibly help it.

Most hospitals provide earphones linked up to the hospital radio system but if you want to take your own transistor radio with you, do make sure this has an ear-piece; other people may want to sleep or may not want to listen to your particular type of entertainment.

Many hospitals admit patients for operations of intermediate severity (and this includes varicose veins) a day before surgery. This enables the surgical staff to check you over thoroughly and give you a full medical examination. The time will also give you the opportunity of meeting the Ward Sister and her nurses (you will soon find out they are just as important as the doctors), learn something about the ward routine and enable you to find your way about. Some hospitals will arrange an early morning admission for an afternoon operation, especially if this is to be done under a local anaesthetic.

Why so many checks?
When you get into hospital you will quickly realize how apt the word 'patient' is – you certainly have to be patient! It seems as if everyone is asking you your name, age, address, name and address of your doctor, next of kin, etcetera, etcetera. This careful routine documentation ensures that your records will be accurately filed; that your doctor will get a report on your stay; and above all, that you will have the correct operation performed! In very rare instances

people have got mixed up in hospital. Not surprising, perhaps, when you realize that hospital theatres may be carrying out twenty, thirty or more operations a day and perhaps there are two or three 'John Browns' and a couple of 'George Smiths' on the list. Nowadays, though, this is almost impossible as each patient is carefully labelled with a plastic name tag, usually around the wrist, on admission. The exact site of the operation is indicated on the patient with an indelible marking pencil (so, in the case of a varicose vein operation, these marks will be placed on the affected leg and perhaps over the particular veins that the surgeon wishes to deal with). The anaesthetist will carefully check your name and details all over again just before the operation, while you are still awake in the anaesthetic room; however tiresome it may seem to the patient, it is a safeguard I thoroughly approve.

Having been documented, you will next be seen by the House Surgeon, whose job it is to give you the complete check-over I mentioned above. He will ask you a lot of questions about your general health and he will examine you from top to toe. Perhaps you

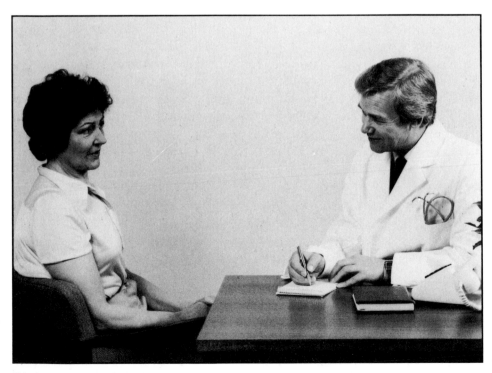

Of the many hospital checks you will have before your varicose veins operation, the most important will be made by the House Surgeon.

will find this rather surprising, possibly even a little embarrassing, when after all you are only bothered about some veins on your leg. Nevertheless this is something you should welcome. I am going to mention some of the things that can imitate the features of varicose veins and their complications in chapter eight and it is just as well to be absolutely certain before surgery that it is your veins, and only your veins, that are the trouble. In addition it is obviously vitally important that a simple operation for varicose veins, which is certainly not essential to life, should be carried out without any risk whatsoever. That is why the House Surgeon is looking for any evidence of recent chest infection or a cold, raised blood pressure, undiagnosed diabetes and so on, all of which might introduce some element of hazard into the anaesthetic and the operation.

You may have had your chest X-rayed at your out-patient visit; if not, it will be done at this stage. A blood test is also usually routine in most hospitals. Many people have a fear of injections – possibly a hangover from childhood when both syringes and needles seemed so huge! But modern needles are very fine (and very sharp) and the House Surgeon or the laboratory technician is very skilled in carrying out the test with the minimum of discomfort.

A specimen of your urine is always taken by one of the nurses and tested for sugar, blood and protein. Again, a very sensible precaution, which occasionally picks up such things as unsuspected diabetes.

If you are admitted to a teaching hospital you will almost certainly have a medical student assigned to you. He (or, in about 50 per cent of cases, she) will have already spent two or three years in medical school, will be keen, intelligent, enthusiastic and dedicated – not the least like some of the characters you see in the various television series! He too will check you over and will be someone to talk to, and someone who will take a great interest and care in your case. I may say that when I was in hospital myself the consultant in charge used me as a specimen to lecture his students about; it certainly helped pass the time and I learned a great deal.

The rest of the time is your own, time to get to know the nurses and the other patients on the ward, and this is where your books and magazines will come in handy.

Preparing for the operation

Either that day, or more usually on the morning of the operation, the area that is to be operated on will have to be completely shaved of all hair. This means, in most varicose veins operations, the whole of the leg (or legs) and the pubic area. Shaving the pubic area can be rather embarrassing for the patient; it is usually carried out by the hospital barber for the men and by one of the nurses for the women. Other hospitals get the patients themselves to do most of the work (Sister will check this to make sure you have made a good job of it) and the disposable safety razors now available are a great help.

The shaving is necessary so that the surgeon can disinfect the skin properly, stitch up the wound without getting bits of hair into it, and get the dressings safely stuck down onto the skin. As the hairs grow back, the area does often feel a little uncomfortable and itchy but there is no way of avoiding this.

Sleeping in a strange bed the night before an operation is not easy, so I advise you not to refuse the sleeping pill that is prescribed; you will benefit from a good night's sleep.

On the morning of your operation you will have to do without your breakfast. Indeed, if you are scheduled for early morning surgery you will be starved of all food and drink from midnight beforehand. If you are on the afternoon operation list you will be allowed an early morning cup of tea or coffee. Keeping you without food is a vital precaution to ensure that your stomach is well and truly emptied by the time you come to have your anaesthetic. This cuts out the risk of vomiting during the introduction of the anaesthetic and means that although you may feel a little nauseated and queasy afterwards, you are very unlikely actually to be sick. You may be worried that you are going to be sick, perhaps as a result of an unpleasant experience many years ago, but with modern anaesthetic techniques it is unusual after this type of surgery.

The anaesthetic

About one and a half hours before your operation, you will receive your pre-medication injection (abbreviated by the hospital staff to 'pre-med'). This usually is given into the tissues of your buttock which are relatively insensitive and a very safe site for injections. The pre-medication has two effects; it makes you feel pleasantly drowsy and free from anxiety (you may even go completely off to sleep) and it also makes your mouth feel very dry; but drying up your secretions is an additional help towards a safe anaesthetic. If you have dentures these are removed, since they could be very dangerous if left in place while you are unconscious.

While you are in this pleasantly dozy state, the theatre porter will collect you on a trolley to take you to theatre. In nearly all hospitals in Britain the operating theatre has an annex, known as the anaesthetic room, where the patient is put to sleep before being taken into the theatre proper. Other countries have different routines, of course; in the United States for instance the patient is usually wheeled directly into the operating room and put to sleep there. British surgeons and anaesthetists think that anaesthetic rooms are a great advantage to the patients, and they are always admired by American surgeons. However, for some reason or another, we cannot seem to persuade the powers that be to introduce them into hospitals in the United States.

The old days of having a mask put over your face to put you to sleep are long past. An almost painless injection into your arm at the elbow or into the back of your hand sends you off into a dreamless sleep within a few seconds.

On waking after your varicose veins operation you will find yourself back in the recovery annex of the operating theatre or tucked up in your own bed on the ward. The wound will certainly feel uncomfortable (many patients describe it as having been kicked on the leg) but this can be relieved quite easily by a post-operative pain-relieving injection. You may feel very slightly nauseated but usually within a few hours you are sitting up in bed and able to enjoy a good drink of water, fruit juice or, best of all, a cup of tea or coffee.

Frequently (some surgeons do this as a routine) the operation is carried out under a local anaesthetic and I have myself used this form of anaesthesia for varicose vein operations on many occasions. The patient may be frightened of going to sleep (just as others are frightened of staying awake!) or may have some slight problem that makes a local anaesthetic preferable and safer. In these circumstances, the pre-operative preparations are very much the same as we have already described, right up to and including the pre-medication injection. Instead of being put to sleep in the anaesthetic room, however, you are taken straight into the operating theatre and feel only one or two pricks in the skin at the sites of the operation. After this you're simply aware that the surgeon is working on your leg – usually it's nothing more than a little discomfort – and indeed many patients doze off and sleep right through it all. Although some surgeons might like an audience, I prefer to put up a screen so the patient cannot watch me.

When you get home

It is rarely necessary for patients to stay in hospital more than a few days after the usual varicose veins operation. Indeed, in many centres the operations are carried out as a day case and the patient returns home on the evening of surgery. Here are a few do's and dont's for you when you reach home.

Dressings   Usually the surgeon will advise you to leave the dressings he has put on untouched until the time comes for the stitches or clips to be removed. This could vary from five to ten days according to the type of operation, the type of stitch used and the particular preference of your surgeon. If you live within reasonable distance of the hospital you will usually be given an appointment to come back to the out-patient clinic or to the ward to have the stitches or clips removed. In other cases the hospital will arrange for your own doctor or for the District or Visiting Nurse to remove them for you, either at home or at the doctor's surgery.

Some hospitals provide an emergency dressing in case the one you have becomes loose or wet. If you do have any kind of problem with the dressing you should let the surgical staff, the Ward Sister or your

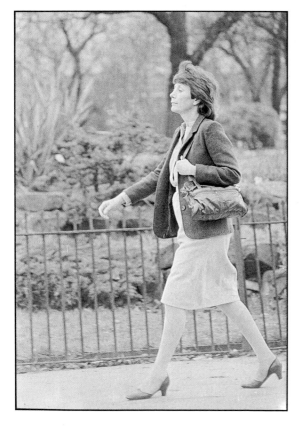

Walking is always good for varicose veins. But after injection treatment or surgery a brisk daily walk in support stockings is essential to prevent the risk of stagnant blood clotting in the leg.

own doctor know at once. Also, if you notice a slight ooze of blood from the wound or a minor discharge, this too should be reported.

Bathing   When your leg has dressings on it and is bandaged, bathing will be a problem. I prefer you to keep the whole area dry and advise that you wash yourself all over, and try to avoid getting the groin region damp. The alternative, if you have a shower available, is to wrap the whole of your leg and groin in a big plastic bag, screwing it up tight above the dressing, and then taking a quick shower.

Walking   With the leg well supported by an elastic stocking, over the bandages at first, the rule is, the more walking you can do the better! Aim at 3 miles (5 km) a day, starting as soon as you get home, but when you're sitting down or lying, prop your leg up in the air.

Sleeping   Prop your leg (or legs) up on pillows so that the heel on the operated side is above the knee and the knee above the hip. This is helped if you have the foot of your bed raised on a firm piece of wood, some bricks or a pile of telephone directories. Elevating your leg will put it in the most comfortable position for the night as well as helping to drain any fluid that might otherwise cause swelling in your leg when you are standing.

Driving   If you live in the middle of the Australian bush, and there is no one else for hundreds of miles around, there is no reason at all why you should not drive your car almost at once. Also if you live in rural parts of America or Britain you should be able to drive as soon as you feel able. Unfortunately, most of us do not live in such idyllic surroundings. Anyone living in or near crowded cities will have experienced other drivers on the road crossing over on the red lights, pedestrians stepping off sidewalks and pavements directly in front of a car and motor cyclists driving the wrong way down one-way streets. All these circumstances mean, of course, that you may have to stamp on the brakes and you can just imagine how difficult that is going to be with a rather uncomfortable incision in the groin and your leg wrapped in bandages. For this reason my advice is not to drive your car in cities or towns until the wound is nicely healed, the stitches are out and the leg is quite comfortable. Usually this is about two weeks after the operation.

Work   This depends almost entirely on what your work happens

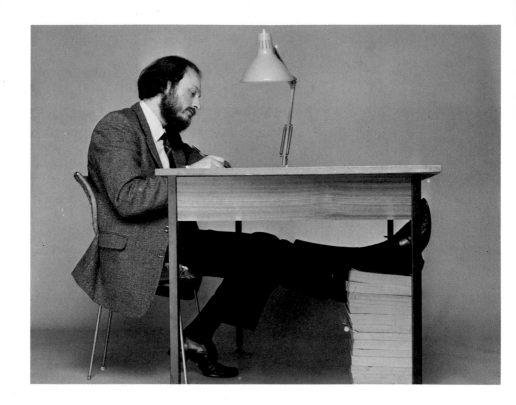

Improvising a method of keeping your leg raised at work – here achieved with telephone directories – will reduce the pressure in your leg veins and aid swift recovery after surgical treatment.

to be. If you can do it sitting at a desk and there is someone to get you to your job and home again, you can be back at work in a very few days indeed (but remember to try and keep your leg raised as much as you can while sitting at the desk, table or work-bench). At the other end of the scale, if you are engaged in heavy manual work, a farmer for example, you will want to have your leg completely healed before getting back to full activity; again this is going to be two or three weeks from the time of surgery. The same restriction applies before you can take up very active sports.

None of these restrictions should be very arduous. Mostly you will be only too pleased to be rid of the troublesome or unsightly veins to risk anything going wrong at this late stage. Unfortunately there is a group of patients who will have to put in a lot of hard work before they can even begin treatment: these, the seriously over-weight, we shall look at next.

6 LOSING WEIGHT TO HELP YOUR VARICOSE VEINS

When an overweight patient comes to see me for treatment of varicose veins or their complications my heart sinks. Obesity has nothing
to do with the development of varicose veins but it does make the
treatment of them very difficult indeed. If injections are needed, the
veins are more awkward to find and we cannot bandage tightly
enough to give the right amount of compression on a leg that's fat
and flabby. If surgery is necessary, the operation is more difficult
when we have to find veins in the depths of fatty tissues, and the
complications of surgery, particularly infection, are always increased.
If the veins have already broken down into an ulcer – bad ulcers are
seen particularly in overweight people – then, again, it is difficult to
compress the leg properly by elastic bandaging and cure is often a
long and tedious business.

I have already stressed the importance of exercise in improving the
muscle-pumping action to return blood from your legs to your heart.
But good long walks, which I have also stressed as an important aid
to getting better, are much more difficult for someone weighing
280 lb (127 kg) say, than for someone around the 100–150 lb (45–
68 kg) mark.

So obesity, with all its other complications, risks and dangers, is
also a serious handicap for the varicose vein sufferer. Weight reduc-
tion is an essential beginning to successful treatment as well as, in
itself, an important step towards improving your general health and
well-being. Indeed, I tell very obese patients that I really cannot get
their legs improved until their weight comes down to a reasonable
level.

Why do some people become overweight?
Fat is the body's principal store of fuel. It is located beneath the
skin, but accumulations are also found within the abdomen, at the
back of the abdominal wall and in the central part of the chest. The
only way to increase this fat store is to take in more food than the
body needs to keep itself going. It is really a matter of simple
arithmetic. If we burn energy at the rate of 2,500 calories a day but

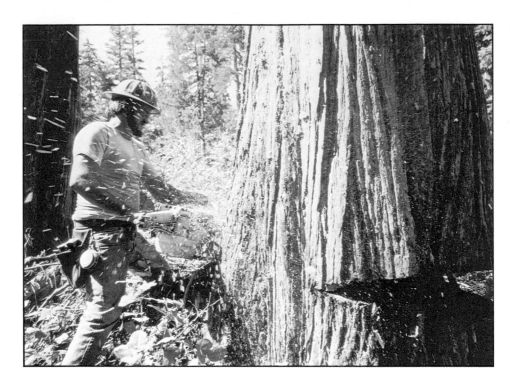

Someone whose job involves strenuous physical activity will need around three times the calorie intake of a sedentary office worker (*opposite*).

have a daily intake of 3,000 calories, the extra 500 calories goes into the fat store. The amount of food required depends on the size of the person and the work that person is doing. A 6 ft 6 in (2 m) Canadian lumberjack will need perhaps three times the calorie intake of a 5 ft 2 in (1.6 m) girl working in a city office. The ideal is to maintain a steady balance between calorie intake and your body's fuel requirement, then your weight will remain steady year in and year out.

Unfortunately, obesity is a plague of modern society. Many people have developed the habit of eating more than they need because eating has now become one of our most important and most enjoyable social habits. Furthermore, our modern life, robbed of much of the physical activity our ancestors were used to, means that we actually need fewer daily calories than ever before. Most of us use some form of motorized transport to take us to work, take the elevator upstairs, in short use every technological convenience to deprive ourselves of the opportunity of burning off those extra calories.

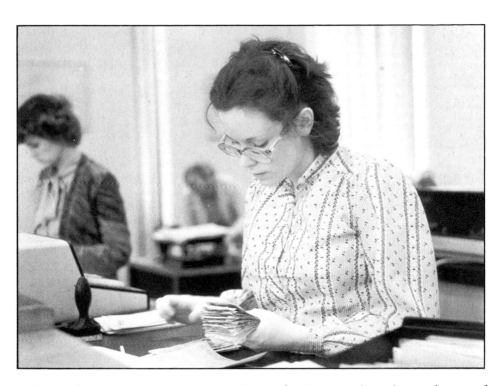

To make matters worse, our diet today is very largely made up of processed foods that are rich in sugar and fat, the latter containing twice the calories of protein or carbohydrates. In former times people ate large amounts of vegetables and grain products (such as unrefined wholewheat bread) which filled their stomachs at a fairly low calorie intake. Today's quick foods (some are more aptly named 'junk foods'), such as bars of chocolate, processed bread, hamburgers and fried potatoes, are low in bulk and high in calories. Furthermore, our alcohol consumption is definitely on the increase and alcohol is very high in calories.

Am I overweight?

First of all you need to know if you are overweight; and if you are, then it is a good idea to have a lower target weight to aim for. The distinction between normal weight and overweight is hard to define precisely, but the table on page 66 is a useful guide to ideal weights for men and women. Although being your ideal weight is excellent as far as your general health and well-being are concerned, the weight at which problems are likely to occur in treatment for your varicose veins is higher than those shown in the table. While it is difficult to be categorical when giving general advice of this kind, it would be fair to say that if you are 15 per cent or more above the weight shown for your height and frame, you would greatly improve your chances of successful varicose vein treatment if you lost some weight. Aim to get down to no more than 10 per cent above your ideal weight.

What can I do to lose weight?

To lose weight is in theory the simplest thing imaginable. If you are overweight then take in fewer calories daily than you require for

Ideal-weight table

Weight table for men of 25 years and over (in indoor clothing)

ft in	Height (cm)	Small frame lb	kg	Medium frame lb	kg	Large frame lb	kg
5 1	(155)	112–120	(51–54)	118–129	(54–59)	126–141	(57–64)
5 2	(157)	115–123	(52–56)	121–133	(55–60)	129–144	(59–65)
5 3	(160)	118–126	(54–57)	124–136	(56–62)	132–148	(60–67)
5 4	(163)	121–129	(55–58)	127–139	(58–63)	135–152	(61–69)
5 5	(165)	124–133	(56–60)	130–143	(59–65)	138–156	(63–71)
5 6	(168)	128–137	(58–62)	134–147	(61–67)	142–161	(64–73)
5 7	(170)	132–141	(60–64)	138–152	(63–69)	147–166	(67–75)
5 8	(173)	136–145	(62–66)	142–156	(64–71)	151–170	(68–77)
5 9	(175)	140–150	(63–68)	146–160	(66–73)	155–174	(70–79)
5 10	(178)	144–154	(65–70)	150–165	(68–75)	159–179	(72–81)
5 11	(180)	148–158	(67–72)	154–170	(70–77)	164–184	(74–83)
6 0	(183)	152–162	(69–74)	158–175	(72–80)	168–189	(76–86)
6 1	(185)	156–167	(71–76)	162–180	(74–82)	173–194	(78–88)
6 2	(188)	160–171	(73–78)	167–185	(76–84)	178–199	(81–90)
6 3	(190)	164–175	(74–80)	172–190	(78–86)	182–204	(83–92)

Weight table for women aged 25 and over (in indoor clothing)
(For women aged between 18 and 25 subtract 1 lb (½ kg) for each year under 25)

ft in	Height (cm)	Small frame lb	kg	Medium frame lb	kg	Large frame lb	kg
4 8	(142)	92–98	(42 44)	96–107	(44–49)	104–119	(47–54)
4 9	(145)	94–101	(43–46)	98–110	(45–50)	106–122	(48–55)
4 10	(147)	96–104	(44–47)	101–113	(46–51)	109–125	(49–57)
4 11	(150)	99–107	(45–48)	104–116	(47–53)	112–128	(51–58)
5 0	(152)	102–110	(46–50)	107–119	(48–54)	115–131	(52–59)
5 1	(155)	105–113	(48–51)	110–122	(50–55)	118–134	(53–60)
5 2	(157)	108–116	(49–53)	113–126	(51–57)	121–138	(55–63)
5 3	(160)	111–119	(50–54)	116–130	(53–59)	125–142	(57–64)
5 4	(163)	114–123	(52–56)	120–135	(54–61)	129–146	(58–66)
5 5	(165)	118–127	(53–58)	124–139	(56–63)	133–150	(60–68)
5 6	(168)	122–131	(55–59)	128–143	(58–65)	137–154	(62–70)
5 7	(170)	126–135	(57–61)	132–147	(60–67)	141–158	(64–72)
5 8	(173)	130–140	(59–63)	136–151	(62–69)	145–163	(66–74)
5 9	(175)	134–144	(61–65)	140–155	(63–70)	149–168	(68–76)
5 10	(178)	138–148	(63–67)	144–159	(65–72)	153–173	(69–78)

fuelling your body. The extra calories will then come from burning your excess store of fat, so every day a little weight will be lost. However, in practice, it can be very difficult and, let's face it, some people find it virtually impossible. Eating is a delightful pastime and to some – the depressed, the lonely, the worried – it is one of the only enjoyments that remains to them. But the benefits of attaining a reasonable weight really are worth making the effort to achieve.

I don't advise crash diets; you may lose weight quickly but you cannot keep them up indefinitely and the relapse rate is high. A steady weight loss, week in and week out, is a much better, wiser and more reliable method.

Fat people often ask me: 'Can't I have some pills or injections to lose weight?' The answer is obvious: only getting your calorie intake below your daily calorie requirement is going to do the trick and that means it is up to you! Of course you'll need encouragement, so ask the rest of the family to co-operate. An excellent idea is to join a local weight-watchers organization; you will soon find you are not the only one with the problem and most people discover that being

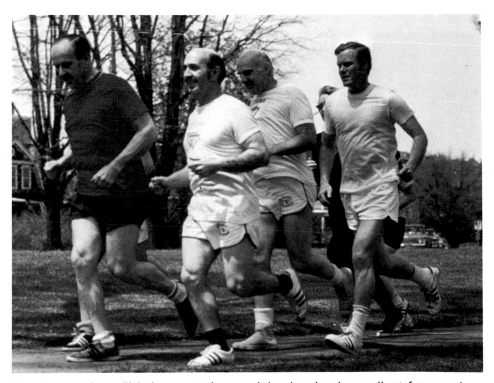

Regular exercise will help you to lose weight. Jogging is excellent for your legs and veins too!

one of a crowd with a united purpose is of tremendous value.

Control the calories

People's calorie requirements differ according to age, sex and activity, but most women will lose weight if they take 1,000–1,200 calories a day. Men, whose calorie requirement is usually higher than women's, often only need to reduce their intake to about 1,500 calories, but everyone varies in this. No-one should habitually take fewer than 1,000 calories a day without close medical supervision, in fact it's not a bad idea to check with your doctor before starting any weight-reducing diet.

The best way to find out the calorie values for foods and drinks is to refer to a calorie-counter booklet, many of which are published by reputable slimming organizations. They are available at most magazine- and bookstores or at your local public library. Either put yourself onto a certain number of calories each day and see how well you lose weight or write down everything you eat for a few days, work out the calorie content roughly and then make yourself a meal plan with about 500 calories fewer per day; again it helps if you enlist the help of your doctor or a dietitian.

The diet you choose must be a sensible one; you could make up a diet where you get 1,200 calories from chocolate and potato chips but it wouldn't keep you healthy for long. So here are a few simple guidelines to follow:

1. Try to eat three meals a day, with small snacks in between if necessary. Scientists have shown that people lose weight better if they eat several small meals a day rather than one huge one.

2. Eat two portions of foods containing high levels of protein (and as little fat as possible) each day. These foods are: lean or white meat, white fish, eggs and low-fat cheese. Pulse vegetables, or legumes, such as cooked dried beans and lentils, are excellent foods, being high in protein and fibre but low in fat.

3. Take ½ pint (1¼ cups)/285 ml of milk (skimmed milk has fewer calories), some low-fat yogurt or a small portion of cheese every day to provide the calcium you need for healthy bones.

4. Have at least 3 slices of wholewheat bread and some cereal, preferably wholegrain, as these are filling and provide fibre.

5. Don't have more than ¾ oz/20 g of fat – butter, margarine, oil or lard, for example – each day; and cut right down on high-fat foods like ice cream and cream sauces. A little fat is essential in your diet but it is very high in calories. Don't fry your food.

6. Cut out high-calorie refined foods such as sugar, chocolate and sweets (candies).

7. Reduce your consumption of alcohol. Better still, cut it out altogether.

8. Make up the rest of your diet with fruit and vegetables. They provide vitamins, minerals and fibre, and are filling yet low in calories.

Making your diet as varied as possible and following these recommendations should keep you healthy while losing weight. If at the same time you can increase the amount of leg exercise you take each day this will help you to lose weight a little faster, stay fit and improve your circulation, thus making treatment of your varicose veins much easier for you and your doctor.

7 IMPROVE THE CIRCULATION IN YOUR LEGS

Leg exercises and elastic support stockings both help you, the varicose vein sufferer, towards the all-important goal of improved blood circulation in your legs. In this chapter I will show you how to use both to your best advantage.

Leg exercises

Exercises for the leg muscles, and raising your legs while at rest, have been repeatedly mentioned as aids to rapid recovery following injection treatment or surgery; as a help during pregnancy; to assist in the healing of ulcers (see page 92); and in general to keep your legs healthy and comfortable.

This section, written with the help of Helen Shilston, physiotherapist at the Westminster Hospital in London, will give you some useful guidelines. It cannot be stressed too often that exercise plays a vital rôle in the treatment of varicose veins, as it helps the muscle pumps of the calves to return blood from the veins in your legs back to the heart. All types of foot and leg exercises are beneficial, as are those carried out in more general pursuits such as walking, swimming, cycling and jogging. In fact, as far as the treatment of varicose veins is concerned, the more activity, the better. Other more vigorous sports such as tennis and squash should be played only when your fitness level permits, and if taking one up for the first time do take it easy to start with.

Exercises to aid circulation
It is a good idea to go through a few simple exercises first thing in the morning to increase your circulation before getting out of bed. You can also do these at other times of the day when you're sitting with your legs elevated, as they do not require a lot of energy.

The following exercise routine (pages 71–4) can be performed before getting up in the morning, as well as during the day.

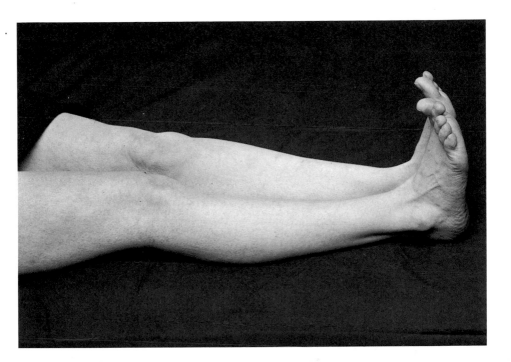

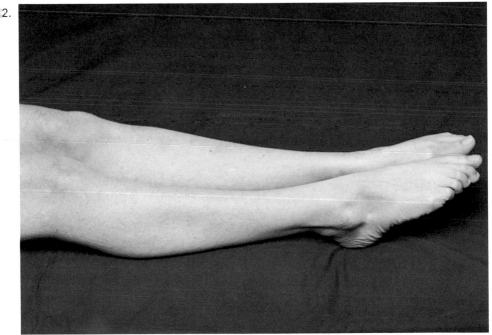

Foot bending   1. Point your feet and toes up towards you as far as you can.   2. Point them down towards the end of the bed. Try to perform this pumping action as vigorously as possible. Repeat ten to fifteen times.

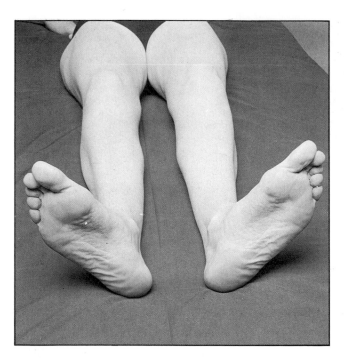

Foot circling Circle your feet from the ankles fifteen times as shown. Then repeat in the other direction.

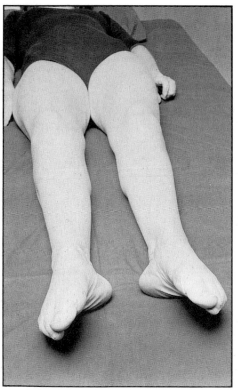

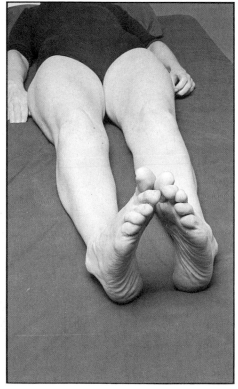

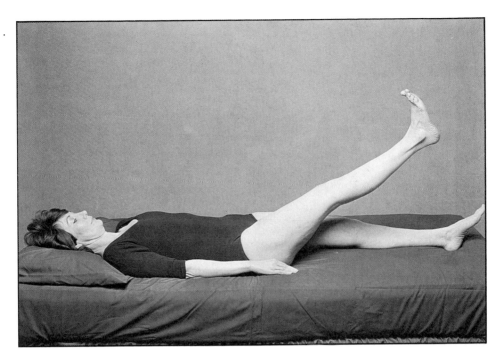

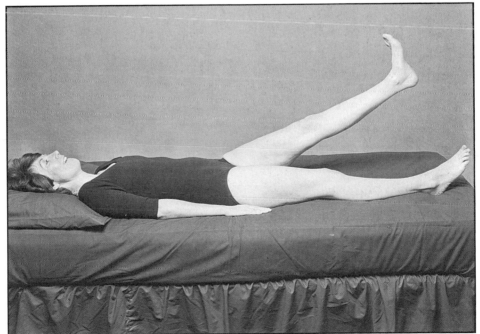

Leg raising 1. With your feet and toes pointing upwards, raise one leg, keeping the knee straight. Hold to the count of three and lower slowly. 2. Repeat with the other leg. Perform sequence twenty times.

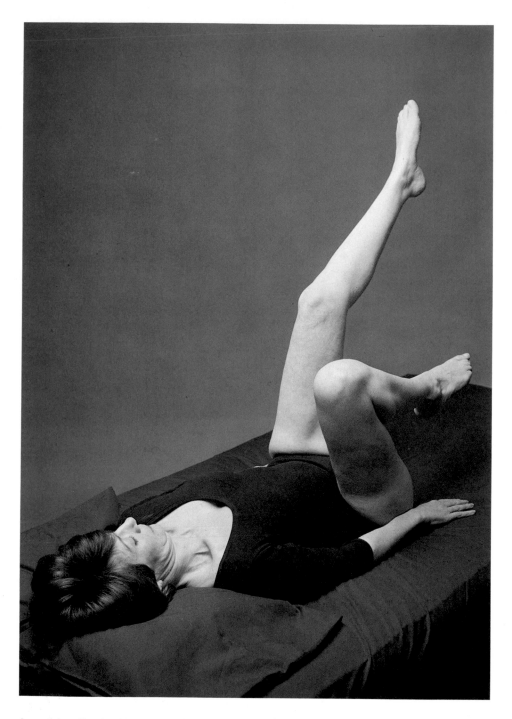

Leg 'bicycling' Alternately bend and stretch your legs in a cycling motion to a slow count of ten. Rest and repeat again as your fitness allows.

Getting out and about

Before getting up in the morning you should put on elastic stockings (see pages 76–81) if you have been told to do so by your doctor, so that you have extra support when you're on your feet. Also it is a good idea to vary (within reason) the height of the heels you wear, so that comfort and good posture are maintained, and the leg muscles are not strained. On no account should you stand around for any length of time. Walking is *the* most important activity and it can be pleasurable too! When you're walking, try not to limp, so that you make the calf muscles work to maximum efficiency in helping your circulation. A stick may be of temporary help if you are having a

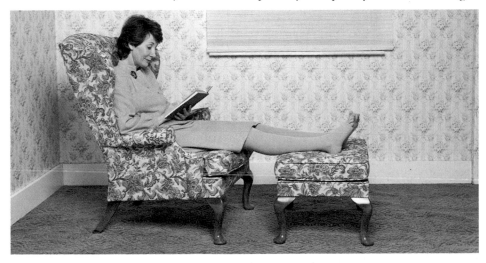

After a long day on your feet, resting in either of these positions, with feet above your hips, will relieve the aching.

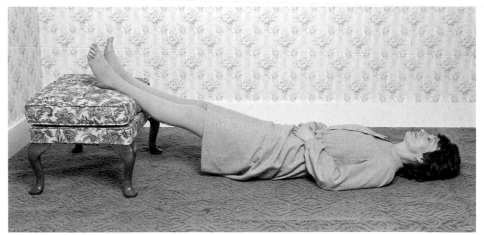

problem with pain or swelling. If you need to go out locally, try walking to the shops, getting off the bus a stop or two before you need to, or parking the car further from your workplace. If you should find walking uncomfortable, try cycling. It may suit you better as there's less weight on your legs, while at the same time you get the right bending and stretching action to improve the circulation.

Daily chores into exercises
Don't think that exercises should be confined to certain times during the day – they can be incorporated into daily routines. For example, housewives who find themselves standing for periods in the kitchen should keep moving by transferring weight from foot to foot, or by stretching up onto tiptoes and down again. Those of you who spend the greater part of your day sitting at desks should rest your legs intermittently on a stool, and frequently change your position by bending and stretching your legs.

At home in the evening it is certainly easier to rest with your legs raised, but it is important not to sit with them crossed as this slows up the blood flow.

If your legs ache, you may find it helpful to lie on your back on the floor with your heels supported on a footstool or chair, or with your feet flat against a wall, heels about 3 ft (1 m) above the floor, so that gravity assists in draining the leg veins.

All these measures will be far more effective if your weight is within normal limits (see page 66), especially as this will reduce strain on the heart and lungs when you exercise. At night, the end of the bed should be raised on blocks. Light bedclothing, such as Continental quilts or loose-fitting blankets, is useful, so that added weight and increased pressure are not put on your legs and feet.

Being sensible about your weight and legs is a continuing process, and once good habits have been introduced, you'll find that exercising and resting with legs raised – possibly, too, the wearing of elastic support stockings, which I am going to discuss next – become a way of life.

Elastic stockings

I have mentioned elastic stockings many times in this book. The reason is that they play an important part in the treatment of varicose veins and their complications. Here, I want to draw together and summarize some important pieces of information about them.

The main purpose of these support stockings is to apply pressure to help the surface veins to do what they've lost the power to do – return the blood into the deep muscle pump of the leg. The stockings are also useful in controlling the swelling of the leg which may result from disease of the veins.

Some uses for elastic stockings

Elastic stockings may be used as the only method of treatment of varicose veins for patients who are old or not well and for whom neither injections nor surgical treatment are advisable. In these cases elastic stockings are not intended as a cure, but they certainly reduce swelling and stop further spreading of the veins. A very good example of this is during pregnancy, when varicose veins can be very troublesome but when active treatment is not advised, either because doctors know that the legs will improve after the baby is born or because doctors are generally reluctant to prescribe treatment that involves interference with the mother's blood circulation system during pregnancy.

Elastic stockings are used both as part of post-operative treatment following surgery and in the after-care of injection treatment. They are also invaluable in the long-term support of the legs after a severe clotting in the deep veins or after a leg ulcer has been healed.

What to look for in a well-designed stocking

A suitable elastic stocking should have the following properties:

1. Open toes – a closed compression stocking is too uncomfortable if the toes are constricted.

2. A stocking should be designed so that compression is greatest at the toes and gradually eases off towards the top of the leg to help maintain a pressure gradient along the leg.

3. The material must be porous to allow evaporation of sweat from the leg.

4. The stocking must be strong enough to apply sufficient compression to the leg. A pressure of less than 30 mm of mercury (mmHg) is of little value and most makes of stockings come in two or three ranges of pressure from 30–60 mmHg. Elastic support tights, for example, although giving some comfort to aching and tired legs have not sufficient compression to

be of long-term value in surgical conditions. However, on special occasions when the appearance of your legs really matters, it is all right to wear support tights, many of which are cosmetically virtually indistinguishable from ordinary tights. Many women find that wearing trousers allows them to look their best, and wear good support stockings at the same time.

Conditions where stockings are inadvisable

Elastic stockings should be prescribed only by a medical practitioner because there are some circumstances in which they can be ineffective or even positively harmful.

1. Legs that are swollen, especially if the leg tissues have watery fluid in them (oedema) due to disease of the veins, should first be raised to reduce the swelling before stockings are put on. However, your doctor must make sure that the swelling is due to the veins, because it may be due to many other causes, such as heart failure, and under such circumstances medical treatment of the patient as a whole is required, not elastic stockings.

2. If there is any associated disease of the arteries to the leg (and in some cases ulceration, which mimics a varicose ulcer – see page 96), then the constricting effect of an elastic stocking can be quite dangerous. A doctor would certainly not prescribe a stocking under such circumstances.

3. If there is an associated severe inflammation of the skin (dermatitis) or an infected ulcer, an elastic stocking is not the right treatment and in any case will rapidly get soaked through with secretions and become unpleasant.

4. Certain groups of people – very old, the infirm, and patients with severe arthritis – will find difficulty in using elastic stockings. Very obese patients also often find them difficult to use and in any case must slim down before they can reap any benefit. Varicose vein sufferers living in a tropical, very humid climate may also find it impossible to use elastic stockings. Indeed, I have had to deal with a number of expatriates who have had to come back to Britain to get their legs cleared up in the more temperate climate for this very reason.

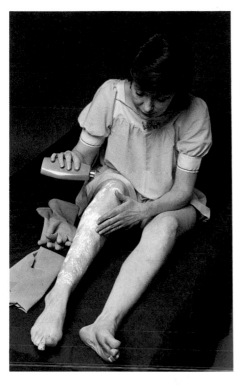

Putting on support stockings

Before getting up in the morning:
1. Apply a little talcum powder to the
leg. 2. Turn stocking inside-out down to
its foot. Then, wearing pimply rubber
gloves, pull foot portion over your
toes. 3. Draw rest of stocking evenly
over the leg, smoothing out all the
creases.

3.

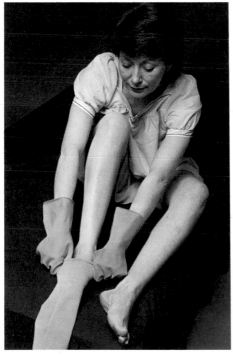

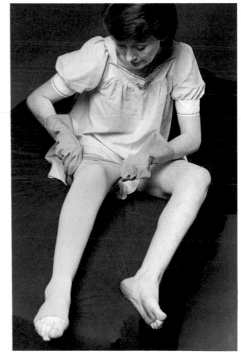

How to put on and take off your stocking

It takes some practice to be able to put on an elastic stocking. A little talcum powder applied to your leg and foot is helpful. If you have a surgical dressing on your leg another tip is to put on an ordinary nylon stocking first. The elastic stocking will glide over this much more easily. Putting your hands in rubber household gloves first is helpful; the friction they create makes it easier for you to pull on your stockings. Use the pimply, rough gloves – not smooth ones. Some brands of stocking supply an anti-slip foot-piece which is put on first and then pulled out once the stocking is in place.

The procedure   First turn the stocking inside out down to its foot; pull the foot portion over your foot, taking great care to smooth it out over the heel; then draw the rest of the stocking evenly over your leg, making sure that you smooth out all the creases. Don't put the stocking on by pulling at the top, but roll it on, bit by bit.

When you want to remove the stocking, your household rubber gloves will again be useful. Hold the stocking at its upper edge and pull downwards towards the heel, turning it inside out as you remove it.

Normally the stocking should be put on first thing in the morning after your leg has been kept raised in bed overnight. It is rarely necessary for you to wear the stocking in bed, provided you keep your leg raised with your heel above your knee and your knee above your hip.

Below-knee stockings will remain in place without any further support (see page 39). If you require above-knee stockings then you will have to wear suspenders to keep them up. Women can use an ordinary suspender belt and men can use either a specially made suspender belt or, less effectively, they can attach the suspender to a button sewn onto the inside of the trouser waistband. Some brands of thigh-length elastic stockings have a waist attachment, which solves the problem of how to keep them up. (See opposite.)

Obtaining and care of the stockings

You can buy elastic stockings without a prescription. Anyone can get a pair by going to a surgical appliance shop or pharmacy and buying them just like any other purchase. However, I have pointed out that it is strongly advisable to wear only stockings that have been prescribed by your medical practitioner or surgeon. In Britain a general practitioner can provide most patients with a prescription for standard elastic stockings. But if the patient is an awkward size or

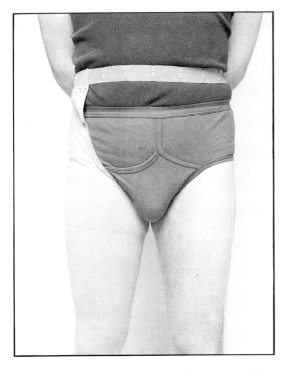

A thigh-length elastic stocking with a waist attachment for men.

shape, he will need stockings such as Sigvaris or Jobst stockings, which require careful measurement of the leg, are more expensive, and are normally prescribed by a hospital consultant.

Having got your prescription, the local hospital appliance department will measure, order and fit the stockings, as well as give you excellent advice about their use and care.

Your elastic stockings should be washed in soap and lukewarm water, rinsed, squeezed out in a towel and then dried flat (not on a radiator). Order two pairs, so that the stockings can be washed daily and used alternately. With reasonable care modern stockings should last for up to six months, although they do gradually stretch. When they have lost much of their elasticity they should be replaced. Most people find that, like ordinary stockings, the heel wears out first.

8 COMPLICATIONS, AND CONDITIONS CONFUSED WITH VARICOSE VEINS

Complications of varicose veins

In a great many cases varicose veins are no more than a nuisance. They are unattractive and they often ache.

Surgeons feel no hesitation in undertaking the treatment of varicose veins purely to improve the appearance of their patient's legs. A typical patient would be, for example, a young woman who enjoys open-air life, swimming and sunbathing, and who finds the presence of the swollen blue veins on her legs an embarrassment.

You may be one of those many sufferers from varicose veins who spend a lot of their time on their feet – such as housewives, shop assistants, postmen and a remarkably high number of nurses and surgeons – and you find that your legs ache and that your ankles become a little puffy at the end of the day. The aching is due to the stretching of the vein wall as it is expanded by blood under pressure in the standing position. The puffiness (or oedema, to give it its correct medical term) is due to the high pressure within the veins which increases the normal movement of fluid across the capillary walls into the soft tissues of the foot and ankle so that the tissues become 'waterlogged'. You will find that both the aching and the swelling will be rapidly relieved when you sit down with your feet raised in the air.

There are, however, a number of complications of varicose veins that, while relatively uncommon, are unpleasant, painful and even, occasionally, dangerous. These are:

1. Phlebitis.
2. Haemorrhage.
3. Pigmentation.
4. Ulceration.

Phlebitis
This is due to a clot forming in the stagnant column of blood in the varicose vein. The clot creates an area of inflammation around it and

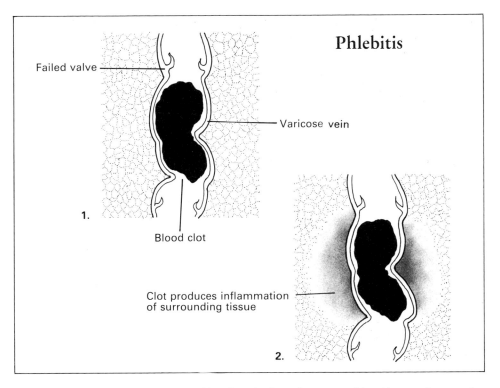

Phlebitis is an inflammation caused by the clotting of stagnant blood in a varicose vein.

in consequence the skin over the clotted part of the vein becomes hot, red, swollen and tender.

Phlebitis occurs only in rather large and chronic varicose veins, so you have no need to worry if you have small, early varicose veins. Indeed, it is not quite such a serious condition as was once thought. In fact, the surgeon who treats varicose veins by injection – which I described in chapter five – is really setting out to produce a controlled localized phlebitis of the vein in order to seal it off.

Patients sometimes fear not only that they may be subjected to a good deal of pain with phlebitis in a surface vein but also that the clot in the vein will become detached and enter the blood circulation system. This does indeed happen when clotting takes place in the *deep* veins of the leg, for example after major operation or injury, but it happens only extremely rarely when phlebitis affects the surface veins of the leg.

How do you know if you have phlebitis? Well, diagnosis is easy, and can be made by you yourself even before coming to the doctor.

The area of redness, pain and tenderness along the vein can be due to no other cause.

Treatment of phlebitis Treatment is simplicity itself. You merely need to rest your leg in the raised position – you can do this either from an armchair, or, preferably, in bed. You'll find light crêpe bandage support comforting and the pain meanwhile can be relieved by suitable pain-relieving pills such as aspirin or paracetamol (acetaminophen).

Although antibiotics are sometimes prescribed for this condition, they are seldom required. They are very useful, indeed they may be life-saving, if you have a disease or wound infected with microbes,

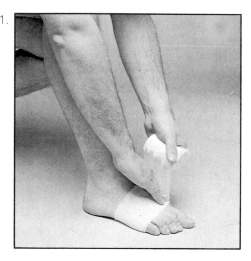

Crêpe support bandaging for phlebitis

1. Tuck the bandage in firmly as you turn it over the foot. Start to unroll it towards the ankle. 2. Cover the heel first by bringing the bandage behind and in front of the heel in a figure of eight.
3. Continue to unroll bandage up the leg until it completely covers the inflamed area. Secure with a safety-pin or Elastoplast.

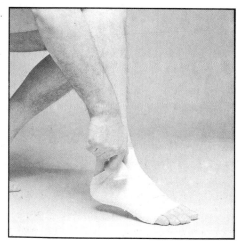

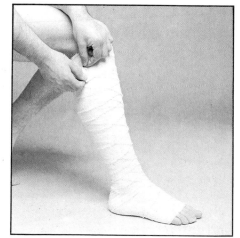

but are quite useless (sometimes positively harmful to people who react against them) when, as in the case of phlebitis, there is no question of bacterial infection. Phlebitis is a chemical inflammation produced by the irritating effect of the blood clot on the surrounding tissues; a similar area of inflammation occurs around a bruise. It is *not* due to bacteria (we call it a sterile inflammatory process).

There is also a good side to phlebitis. Just as a surgeon produces a localized chemical inflammation in a varicose vein to cure it by injection treatment, so quite often after an attack of phlebitis the varicose veins settle down and become less prominent than before. I agree that it's not the ideal treatment but at least it is a little comfort to the phlebitis sufferer to think that the leg may look rather better after the attack than it did before.

Haemorrhage

Haemorrhage, or bleeding, is one of the complications that comes to the mind of the layman, sufferer and non-sufferer alike, when seeing badly swollen veins. In fact, this potentially dangerous complication is unusual, and occurs only in particularly large and particularly prominent veins that lie immediately below the skin of the ankle or the lower calf. Sometimes these enormous veins seem to have only a paper-thin layer of skin between them and the surface of your leg. If you injure one of these veins – it can take only a trivial matter such as a knock getting in or out of a bus or car, or even just scratching an itch in the overlying skin – there can be a serious gush of blood from the opened vein if you're standing up. This gush is due to the fact that, as we have already discussed at some length, pressure in these veins is very high when you are in the standing position and represents the pressure of the column of blood stretching all the way down from your heart to your ankle.

Do's and don'ts Like the treatment for phlebitis, treatment for haemorrhage too is simple: the high pressure within the vein is relieved by lying down and holding your leg in the air. A firm bandage should be applied (a clean handkerchief will serve just as well) and the emergency is over. (See page 86.) Trying to improvise a tourniquet around the leg is worse than useless because, if this is put on by an amateur, it actually increases the pressure within the vein and the bleeding becomes still fiercer.

I shall never forget how, as a young doctor, I treated a woman who had injured her varicose vein and had been brought into hospital sitting in a cab. Her sitting position, of course, did nothing to

85

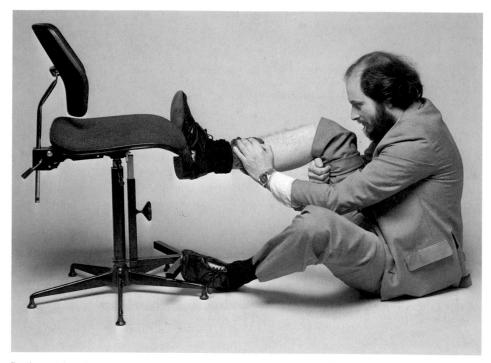

Profuse bleeding from a varicose vein can be dangerous. To stop it, simply raise your foot and apply a clean handkerchief or cloth firmly to the bleeding area with the palm of your hand.

prevent the high-pressure bleeding and she was all but dead on arrival. Only a prompt blood transfusion in the Casualty Department saved her life. If only that cab driver had learned a little first aid, he would have done her a great service (as well as preventing the inside of his cab from being ruined) merely by bringing her into hospital with her leg lifted up onto the seat in front!

Varicose pigmentation
Many patients fear the development of these next two complications – the discolouration of areas of the leg, known as pigmentation, and the open sores of ulceration. There was once some cause for these fears, because they used to be extremely common but now, with improved health services and surgical facilities, these very advanced forms of varicose veins that we used to see often in our hospital clinics are fortunately becoming much rarer.

Pigmentation has all sorts of names – including varicose pigmentation, varicose eczema, gravitational pigmentation and varicose dermatitis. Just why this unsightly skin discolouration comes about can

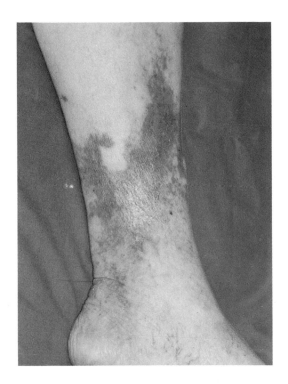

Varicose pigmentation – also called varicose eczema or dermatitis – can be camouflaged with skin-coloured cosmetic creams.

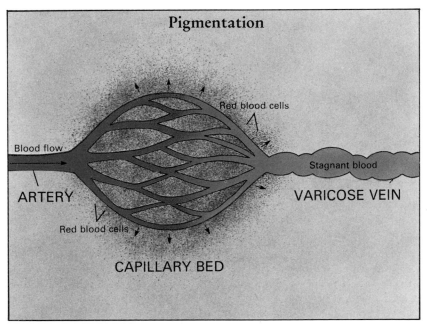

Stagnant blood in a varicose vein forces the red blood cells out through the delicate capillaries and into the skin, resulting in pigmentation.

easily be explained. Once again, it is the result of high pressure present within the varicose vein. This is transmitted right down to the thin-walled capillaries of the lower leg and forces the red blood corpuscles through them into the surrounding soft tissues of the skin. The red cells break down into an iron-containing pigment called haemosiderin, and it is this substance that gives the bluish-brown pigmentation so characteristic of this condition.

Once badly pigmented, the skin will not return to its normal appearance, although any further pigmentation can be prevented if the underlying veins are treated. Sometimes the appearance of the leg can be improved if the doctor can treat the complication in its early stage, and skin-coloured cosmetic creams are available which effectively camouflage the discolouration.

Ulceration

In an advanced case of varicose veins, the skin of the lower leg becomes pigmented, thin and poorly nourished. It is poorly nourished because the high pressure in the varicose veins prevents arterial blood and its oxygen and nutrients from being pushed through the fine network of capillaries to supply the skin (see page 87). At this stage a minor injury, sometimes merely scratching the irritating skin, is all that may be necessary to cause the development of an ulcer. In a healthy leg an injury such as this would heal within a day or two. With the skin starved of nourishment and the blood's healing properties, the tiny wound breaks down into an ulcer, which may take several weeks of careful treatment to heal. If the ulcer is neglected it may enlarge and become a painful, burdensome misery to its owner.

Prevention is better than cure Varicose ulcers are always preceded by at least several years of slowly worsening trouble with the leg, leading to pigmentation, itchiness and often very prominent and unpleasant varicose veins. If you can let your doctor begin treatment at this pre-ulcer stage so that he can deal with the veins, then ulceration will be prevented. The steps he will advise will be:

1. Support the leg with elastic stockings.
2. Elevate the leg in bed at night.
3. Exercise regularly.
4. Lose weight if overweight.
5. Take care not to scratch or injure the threatened skin of the leg.

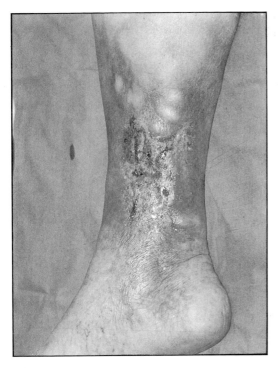

A leg ulcer like this can be prevented by taking the simple steps outlined opposite. If one does develop, the treatment is simple but effective: keep the leg raised and supported by elastic bandaging (see overleaf).

As in so many situations, this prevention is far, far better than what may turn out to be a long, tedious and painful cure.

Small ulcers If the skin does break down into an ulcer following some slight damage to your leg such as a knock or scratch, the earlier you can get to your doctor for efficient treatment the better. Indeed, a small ulcer can be completely healed within a very few weeks.

The large nasty-looking ulcers that we see in our hospital clinics from time to time always result either from neglect of a small ulcer, or from its inappropriate or inadequate treatment.

Treatment of varicose ulcers

To cure an ulcer we have to deal with the cause – the poor blood supply to the skin of the affected area due to the high pressure in the draining veins – which means emptying the high-pressure veins. This is done by two combined measures: elevating the leg and supporting it with elastic bandaging.

Elevation When you raise your leg it empties the veins of blood by means of gravity. If you keep your heel above your knee and your knee above your hip while in bed, you will have achieved a great deal already towards healing the ulcer. You can elevate the leg either by using pillows under the leg or by placing blocks under the foot of the bed to raise it 12 in (30 cm) in the air.

Of course, keeping your leg up for eight to ten hours at night during the sleeping period is easy enough, and you can add to the good work by putting your leg up whenever possible when sitting down during the day. It is a fact, though, that most people just don't relish the prospect of remaining in bed with their leg elevated for several weeks continuously, even though this alone will get the ulcer to heal in the great majority of cases.

Elastic bandaging   You are probably one of the many people with a busy household to run or a living to earn and so must be able to walk about during the day. This means that we must use our second means of treatment for varicose ulcers, firm elastic bandaging (which compresses the surface veins more tightly than elastic stockings). This squeezes the blood out of the incompetent surface veins, through perforators, or linking veins, and into the deep veins of the leg. Then when you walk, these veins will be emptied actively back towards the heart through the pumping action of the muscles of your leg, thus greatly improving the tissue-nourishing circulation of blood around the ulcer.

There are two types of elastic support bandage available. One is strong elasticated web bandage that can be wound around the leg each day from the toes to just below the knee. It requires a great degree of skill to obtain a firm constant pressure along the leg. Although it is a highly effective type of support, most patients (or their families) lack the expertise needed to carry out this kind of bandaging satisfactorily.

The majority of patients, therefore, must have their leg supported by the elasticated adhesive tape known in Britain as Elastoplast. This can be applied by a nurse or doctor in an out-patient clinic or in your general practitioner's surgery, and renewed every couple of weeks. Only an elastic bandage or Elastoplast will do – crêpe bandages or support stockings simply lack the elastic strength required for the job of emptying the veins and are quite ineffective in helping an ulcer to heal.

Unfortunately, many people are, or become, sensitive to Elastoplast, and the discoloured, scaly skin around the ulcer seems especially prone to such an allergy. Obviously, a sensitivity rash is the very last thing you want to have in this condition.

Having an ulcer bandaged

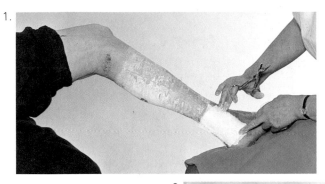

Half-way through treatment, this patient is having his leg rebandaged. A piece of sterile gauze has been placed over the ulcer on the inner side of the ankle. This is held in place with a sticky Viscopaste bandage.

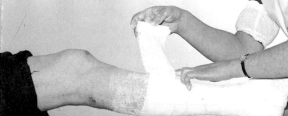

The Viscopaste bandage is applied smoothly from the toes to below the knee.

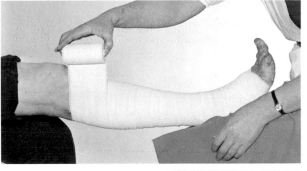

Elastoplast is now used to bandage over the Viscopaste. This requires considerable skill to ensure smooth application.

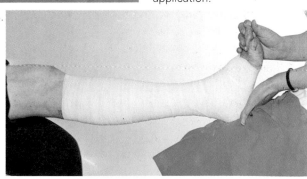

The procedure is now complete.

How to guard against adhesive-tape allergy   If you do suffer from such an allergy then tell your doctor or nurse and they will protect your skin from direct contact with the Elastoplast by placing a pad of ordinary dry sterile gauze over the ulcer itself and then wrapping the leg in a simple gauze bandage before bandaging your leg firmly and smoothly with Elastoplast from the toes to just below the knee. The method is shown in the series of illustrations on page 91.

One problem with the gauze bandage is that it has a tendency to wrinkle as the Elastoplast is wrapped over it. For this reason in many clinics some type of proprietary adherent bandage (such as Ichthopaste, Coltapaste or Viscopaste in Britain) is used next to the skin. Certainly this makes the smooth application of the Elastoplast an easier task for the doctor or the nurse.

Exercise and losing weight   With the leg firmly bandaged, it is up to you to use the muscle pump. This means active walking exercises – a good brisk 3 miles (5 km) a day as a minimum.

All too often, varicose ulcer sufferers tend to be overweight. This makes compression of the leg veins difficult and being fat makes active exercise more of a problem than it should be. A reducing diet (see chapter six) for such patients is a really important first step towards effective treatment.

So, to sum up the requirements in treating a varicose ulcer, we have these four points to observe:

1. Elevation of the leg at night.
2. Skilled elastic bandaging.
3. Active exercises.
4. Weight watching.

Ointments, creams and lotions   Some readers, I am sure, will be very surprised to find no mention of some special ointment, lotion, salve, cream, impregnated gauze, antibiotic or steroid that I recommend as absolutely essential to clean up and heal the ulcer. The reason for this is very simple – none of them works! Indeed, my first duty when I have to deal with a large, obstinate, unhealed, angry-looking ulcer, surrounded by an intense itchy inflammation of the skin is to persuade my reluctant patient to throw away all the pots, tubes, bottles and packets that have been used to date and to adopt the inexpensive simple routine outlined above.

It is very often the sensitivity of the skin to these various medicaments that is actually prolonging the problem and preventing the firm, continuous, active support of elastic bandaging: the essential basis of effective treatment.

Although the ulcer itself may be nasty, smelly and infected, the base of the ulcer is in fact a very effective barrier to bacteria invading the surrounding tissues, so antiseptics and antibiotics are just not needed. Doctors very rarely have to prescribe antibiotics for infection spreading from an ulcer, but if this does occur we use a short course either of injections or else pills by mouth, and *never* anything applied directly to the ulcer or its surrounding area.

Once the ulcer begins to heal, we can deal with the underlying varicose veins that so often also need to be treated. As I have explained in chapter five these can be injected if they are confined to the calf but when it is a case of large varicose veins in the thigh and at the groin, surgery will be necessary to clear them.

Long-term precautions

Getting the ulcer healed and dealing with the underlying veins are only phases one and two; phase three is vitally important. If you have suffered from an ulcer, it means, as I have pointed out, that severe damage is present in the vein system of the leg. Constant vigilance will be essential in the future. This means a life-time of elastic stocking support when up and about – not really a great burden, since modern elastic stockings are comfortable and look good (see page 39); a life-time of sleeping with your leg or legs raised in bed at night; and, just as important, keeping up the excellent habit of active walking, as well as a careful watch on any tendency to put on weight.

Remember that it takes only a minor injury to bring about ulceration, so that it is important to care for your legs as a mother cares for her baby. The reward is well worth while: the prevention of a further troublesome spell of treatment for a new ulcer.

Leg ailments sometimes confused with varicose veins

Spider veins (telangiectases)

It is quite common for women to have tiny swollen veins in their upper legs and lower thighs; they are seen less often in men. They seem to occur early in pregnancy, which suggests that they may have something to do with the effects of the sex hormones circulating in

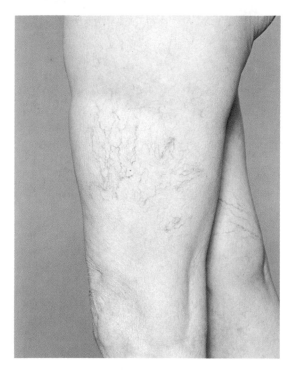

Spider veins are not related to varicose veins. They are harmless and require no treatment.

the bloodstream. These little marks are simply tiny visible veins in the skin; they have nothing to do with varicose veins although many people with these spider veins also have varicose veins. They are given all kinds of other names, including capillary veins, burst veins, venous starts, spider naevi and telangiectases.

Women are often very self-conscious about these skin blemishes but I have always personally advised against any treatment for them. Some surgeons do use injection treatment (similar to that used in treating ordinary varicose veins), others use heat treatment (diathermy) or destroy the veins by electric needles (electrolysis). Although these methods may be successful, they may also fail, in which case they could leave a brownish discolouration of the skin that may be worse than the original blemish. These veins do not spread or get worse and they are not related to varicose veins. As they are also completely harmless, I personally feel that the patient is best advised just to forget about them or to disguise them with skin make-up. There are some extremely effective modern camouflage cosmetics on the market.

Other causes of pain in the leg
It is true that prominent varicose veins can cause aching and discom-

fort in your legs when you have been standing for a long time, but the aching can have other causes such as sciatica, arthritis, obstruction in a leg artery, or muscle cramps.

Sciatica   is often due to a displacement of one of the discs between the vertebrae in the lower spine. When this happens pain spreads down the back of the leg. It is usually much more severe than the ache of varicose veins and does not disappear as soon as you raise your leg in the air – an action that immediately relieves the congesting discomfort that comes with varicose veins. Doctors do this 'straight leg test' to find out whether the aching in their patient's leg is due to varicosities or to sciatica.

Arthritis of the knee   is common in plump, middle-aged and elderly women. The knee crackles and is painful when it is moved.

Arterial disease is a common fact of life as we get older and is usually the result of arteriosclerosis – thickening of the artery walls. It is particularly marked where there is a strong association with a lifetime of cigarette-smoking. One of the typical symptoms of this disease is a pain in your calf after you've been walking a certain distance, perhaps 100–200 yd (90–180 m); you will find you have to stand still for several minutes before the pain goes away. You will then be able to walk a similar distance before the pain starts up again. When your doctor examines you, he will find that the foot you complain of is cooler than the rest of your body (arterial blood circulating through the skin gives out warmth), and he will also find that the pulses in the leg below the constricted artery cannot be detected. This will indicate to him that you have arterial disease.

Muscle cramps   These spasms, when the muscles contract very tightly cause severe pain and often occur at night. The agonizing pain lasts for only a few seconds, although it seems much longer to the victim. As far as I know, no-one has any explanation for this condition or any rational suggestion for its treatment.

Many people with these and other painful conditions of their legs may have some small varicose veins as well. In contrast, many people with quite large varicose veins may have no symptoms at all apart from the unsightly appearance of their legs.

   What you should not do is always to attribute pain in your legs to the varicose veins. You are then likely to be very distressed, and quite rightly so, if the pain remains after the varicose veins have been treated in the mistaken notion that they were the prime cause of your troubles.

Ulcers of the leg

We know that a very high proportion of ulcers of the leg are due to varicose veins. However, it is very important not to overlook the more unusual causes of a leg ulcer.

After varicose veins the most common cause of ulceration of the leg, and this amounts to perhaps 5 per cent of all the patients we see, is insufficient blood supply from the *arteries*. The reason for this is usually arteriosclerosis (thickening of the arteries) and it is almost always found in heavy smokers. These patients may also be suffering from varicose veins, of course, and unless the doctor looks carefully for evidence of arterial disease (a cold foot with poor circulation and a lack of pulses in the leg) he may well think that the ulceration is due entirely to the obvious varicose veins.

Injury is another cause of an unhealed ulcer on the leg. Again, this is commonly seen in elderly patients. The combination of a nasty injury to the leg and the lack of any evidence of vein disease makes this type of ulcer quite obvious in most cases.

9 QUESTIONS AND ANSWERS

If you or someone in your family has varicose veins, I hope this book will have given you a better understanding of what varicose veins are and what you can do about them. I also hope it will have removed some of your doubts and fears about them.

In this last chapter I want to gather together some of the questions that doctors and nurses are frequently asked about varicose veins and which, though they have been dealt with more fully in the course of the book, those of you who would like a quick answer may find useful.

What are varicose veins?
They are twisted, swollen, bluish veins lying just below the skin of the leg. They can be seen clearly when you stand, but if you lie down and put your leg up in the air, the veins empty and usually disappear. Their unsightliness is one of the most frequent reasons why people want them treated, but apart from their appearance, they also cause aching pain in the legs and if neglected may develop unpleasant complications, which include eczema, discolouration, ulceration of the skin, thrombosis and haemorrhage.

Why do people get varicose veins?
The simple answer is that in the majority of cases we just do not know. The normal superficial veins of the leg have an efficient system of valves that direct the blood back to the heart. The underlying cause of varicose veins is undoubtedly failure of these valves, which then permit blood to flow backwards in the veins of the leg at high pressure. We know that varicose veins run in families so there would appear to be an inherited factor which may be some congenital defect in the valves, especially when varicose veins develop in adolescents or young adults. In other cases, the damage to the valves may result from an injury or from thrombosis (clotting) in the deep veins of the leg – something which may follow a surgical operation, a prolonged illness or occasionally childbirth.

Do tight garters cause varicose veins?

There is no evidence that tight garters, constricting clothes or prolonged standing *cause* varicose veins. However, if you already have
varicose veins then there is no doubt that anything which raises the
pressure in your veins such as tight clothing or prolonged standing
will make the veins distend and ache. For your own comfort, therefore, these should be avoided.

Does smoking cause or aggravate varicose veins?

Although I strongly advise my patients not to smoke, because of the
undoubted links between cigarette smoking and lung cancer, chronic
bronchitis and arterial disease, there is no connection between smoking and either the origin of varicose veins or the aggravation of
varicose veins that are already there. However, I would not like
anybody to take this as an excuse for continuing the habit!

Should I take the contraceptive pill if I have varicose veins?

Women with varicose veins are definitely at a slightly greater risk of
developing clotting (or thrombosis) on the pill than women with
normal legs. This risk is especially so over the age of about thirty-
five. If you have severe varicose veins your doctor will probably
advise against the pill and recommend some other form of contraception. Once the veins have been adequately treated, however, the
pill can be prescribed quite safely.

Does pregnancy cause varicose veins?

Many women attribute their varicose veins to pregnancy. Indeed,
varicose veins often become obvious early on in pregnancy. The
oestrogen hormone level is raised in the blood during pregnancy and
this undoubtedly has the effect of relaxing and so distending the
veins. Moreover, the pressure of the enlarging womb presses on the
pelvic veins and raises the pressure within the leg veins that drain up
into them. Very likely pregnancy does not actually cause varicose
veins, but if you have a tendency to varicose veins they are undoubtedly going to become worse during pregnancy and also during subsequent pregnancies. Another related problem, which is almost
unique to pregnancy, is the development of varicose veins on the
vulva, around the entrance to the vagina. Although these can be
quite uncomfortable and unsightly, they nearly always disappear
shortly after the birth of the baby.

How are varicose veins treated during pregnancy?

Most doctors are very conservative. You can keep your legs comfortable by wearing elastic support stockings. You should rest your legs in the elevated position during the day and learn to sleep with your legs elevated in bed. Avoid standing; but walking exercises are excellent. The veins may improve remarkably once your baby is delivered; if they do not, then more active treatment either by injections or surgery may be required. Unfortunately, if you have vein trouble in one pregnancy you are likely to get it in the next, but by taking early precautions, support stockings, elevation and exercise, your symptoms can be kept under control.

Can elastic support stockings cure varicose veins?

Unfortunately, no. A well-fitting pair of elastic stockings are invaluable for those who are not fit enough or who are unwilling to undergo more extensive treatment for their veins. Elastic stocking support is what we call a palliative: in other words, it relieves symptoms by compressing the varicose veins, but it certainly does not cure them. Elastic stockings are very helpful in the follow-up treatment after surgery or injections for varicose veins and are also extremely useful in relieving the symptoms of varicose veins during pregnancy.

Which is better: injection treatment or surgery?

Injection treatment and surgery are not rivals, since each method has its own applications. Indeed, it is not uncommon for both methods to be used in the same patient. The injections work by producing a small area of inflammation in the wall of the vein which will then become sealed off with scar tissue, thus obliterating the varicose vein. It is a very useful treatment in dealing with the common problem of fairly small veins below the knee and around the calf. Surgery is usually required for more extensive varicose veins that extend up to the thigh and the groin. Afterwards, it may be necessary to inject any remaining varicose veins lower down the leg. Injection treatment is also very useful in dealing with small recurrences which may occur after surgical treatment.

What are the advantages and disadvantages of each method?

Injection treatment is given on an out-patient basis, so there is no need to be admitted to hospital or to have an anaesthetic. If the veins are not all cleared up, the injections can be repeated and if further varicose veins develop at a later stage these too can be cleared up by further injections. Occasionally a small area of brown discolouration may occur at the site of the injection and, rarely, there may be a tiny ulcer at the injection site if any of the injection material has escaped under the skin. The ulcer will heal quite quickly with simple dressings.

Surgical treatment requires admission to hospital, if only as a 'day-case', and either a general or local anaesthetic. As with any other operation, there is always the possibility of bleeding in the wound or of infection, even though these risks are nowadays very slight indeed.

What is the risk of recurrence of varicose veins after treatment?

Unfortunately something like 20 per cent of vein sufferers are likely to develop further varicose veins following treatment. In some cases this is because veins that have been injected have swollen again or one of the veins that was not tied off surgically gradually expands. More often these veins represent new varicosities which have developed as further valves become faulty. However, the development of further varicose veins is quite a slow process and further injections or quite minor surgery can deal with these new veins effectively.

Is clotting in my varicose veins dangerous?

Thrombosis in the *deep* veins of the leg (not the ones which become varicose) is a complication that occasionally follows major surgery, prolonged bed-rest from illness or, rarely, pregnancy. In this condition there is indeed a small risk that the clot may detach and lodge in the lung (pulmonary embolism). Clotting in the varicosed superficial veins of the leg, called phlebitis, (see question below) is so rarely accompanied by this complication that it can pretty well be ignored. So, the answer to this question is no!

What is phlebitis?

The stagnant column of blood within very swollen varicose veins may clot and set up a localized area of inflammation. The segment of affected surface vein becomes hot, red, swollen and tender. It is very rarely due to a bacterial infection and therefore does not require antibiotic treatment. If you are found to be suffering from phlebitis you will be advised to go to bed and rest your leg in the elevated position, with the heel above the knee and the knee above the hip. The whole affair will then settle down quite quickly.

What are my chances of developing a varicose ulcer?

If you have minor varicose veins and these are treated, there is not much risk of you developing an ulcer. Ulcers usually develop in legs that have long-established varicose veins and already have patches of inflamed skin known as varicose eczema. Anyone who has had a thrombosis of the deep veins of the leg and who has a swollen and discoloured leg as a result is also at risk. Ulceration usually occurs in such legs as a result of a minor accident, so you should be particularly careful about keeping your legs out of harm's way.

How can I get my varicose ulcer healed?

The treatment of a varicose ulcer is basically simple. Your leg should be supported by an elastic bandage which will compress the affected veins and assist their returning blood from the leg to the heart. Once your leg is effectively bandaged, you are encouraged to take active walking exercises so that the blood in the veins is returned through the muscle pump of the leg. Drainage is also helped by elevating your leg at night in bed, by avoiding standing and by keeping your leg elevated when you're sitting down. There is no need to apply any ointments, salves or antibiotics; indeed, the sensitivity of the skin to these often only makes the ulcer worse. If you are overweight this will make the efficient bandaging of the legs difficult and will make active exercising harder so that you will need to go on a strict weight-reducing diet before treatment can be really effective.

Can I stop varicose veins from developing?

Unfortunately, at present we know of no way of doing this. However, early treatment of varicose veins, either by injection or by surgery, is highly effective and has a very good chance indeed of stopping you developing the complications of this condition. If you have varicose veins, you can help the surgeon immensely by a few simple common-sense measures: avoid standing; learn to keep your legs raised when you are sitting down or lying in bed; take plenty of active exercise to keep the muscles of your legs pumping the blood back to your lungs; and keep slim!

ACKNOWLEDGEMENTS

The publisher would like to thank the following individuals and organizations for their permission to reproduce photographs: Thompson/Miller Services, Toronto (page 38); NFB Photothèque, Ottawa (pages 23, 27, 36, 64, 65 and 67); The Photographers' Library, London (page 26); Adrian Pope, London (page 56); Westminster Medical School's Photographic Department (pages 10, 19, 42, 43, 87, 89, 91 and 94).

The diagrams on pages 13, 14, 15, 16, 18, 20, 24, 35, 45, 50, 51, 83 and 87 were drawn by David Gifford.

The photographs on pages 25, 39, 47, 60, 62, 71–5, 79, 81, 84 and 86 were taken by Dave Brown and Dave Robinson.

Finally, thanks are due to Helen Shilston and Sister Hunt of Westminster Hospital for their expert advice during the studio photography; to Julia Drake for modelling many of the studio photographs; and to Parker Knoll Furniture Ltd for the loan of the Bosworth chair and footstool appearing on page 75.

INDEX

37, 40, 99; putting on and taking off, 80–1
Elastoplast, 90–2
electrolysis, 94
exercise, 8–9, 30–1; after injection therapy, 48, 49; to improve circulation, 70–6; and leg ulcers, 92; and obesity, 63; in pregnancy, 37

Fegan, George, 37, 44, 45
female sex hormones, *see* hormones
femoral vein, 17, 50–1
fibre, in diet, 29–30, 68–9

garters, 9, 25, 37, 98
genetics, 27, 97
gravitational pigmentation, *see* pigmentation

haematoma, 52
haemorrhage, 31, 82, 85–6, 97
haemosiderin, 88
heart, physiology, 12–13
heart attacks, 33
heart failure, 78
heat, and varicose veins, 24, 78
heat treatment, spider veins, 94
heredity, 27, 97
high blood pressure, 57
hormones, contraceptive pills, 32, 33; during pregnancy, 35, 98; effects on veins, 19, 24, 31, 33, 98
hospitals, 54–60; *see also* surgery
housework, 76

iliac veins, 30
inflammation, injection treatment, 44–5
inherited factors, 27, 97

injection treatment, 41–6, 52–3, 99–100; complications, 48–9; follow-up care, 46–8; obese patients, 63; permanency, 48; in pregnancy, 36–7; spider veins, 94; vulval varicosities, 38
intestines, diverticular disease, 29
iron chloride, 41

jogging, 8, 70

knees, arthritis, 95

legs, arterial disease, 95; circulation of blood in veins, 16–17; exercise, 8–9, 70–6; non-varicose ulcers, 96; pain in, 76, 94–6; raising, 9, 37, 41, 61, 76, 89–90; sciatica, 95
lifestyle, 28–31

men, varicose veins, 31
menstruation, 35
muscles, and circulation of blood in veins, 16–17; cramps, 34, 95; exercises, 70–6

obesity, 9, 40, 46, 63–9, 92, 101
oedema, 78, 82
oestrogen, contraceptive pills, 32, 33; effects on veins, 24, 31, 33, 98; in pregnancy, 24, 98
ointments, leg ulcers, 92–3, 101
operations, 49–53, 54–9; post-operative care, 59–62, 77

pain, in legs, 94–6
pain-relievers, 48, 52, 59, 84
paracetamol, 48, 52, 84
perforating veins, 17, 20, 90;

Other books in the
Positive Health Guide
Series

THE BACK – RELIEF FROM PAIN
Dr Alan Stoddard

Hope at last for the millions who suffer back pain! Dr Stoddard explains how the back works and what to do when it lets you down.

DON'T FORGET FIBRE IN YOUR DIET
Dr Denis Burkitt

This world-renowned medical scientist presents the first wide-ranging survey on the importance of fibre in preventing many typically western diseases.

BEAT HEART DISEASE!
Dr Risteard Mulcahy

A reassuring look at one of today's most serious 'epidemics' – showing how changes in lifestyle could dramatically reduce the occurrence of heart disease and stroke.

OVERCOMING ARTHRITIS
Dr Frank Dudley Hart

A leading rheumatologist describes just what arthritis and rheumatism are, and includes a wealth of ideas on how to keep your joints as supple and pain-free as possible.

ASTHMA AND HAY FEVER
Dr Allan Knight

Breathing difficulties or a streaming nose afflict thousands every year. Here an expert allergist explains what is happening to you and what you can do to ease the problems.

PSORIASIS
Dr Ronald Marks

This is one of the commonest skin diseases, affecting hundreds of thousands each year. Here at last is a book that answers everyone's questions.

HIGH BLOOD PRESSURE
Dr Eoin O'Brien & Prof Kevin O'Malley

Written by two eminent physicians, this is a comprehensive and practical guide to detecting, preventing and controlling high blood pressure.

THE HIGH-FIBRE COOKBOOK
Pamela Westland
Introduced by Dr Denis Burkitt

This book combines the healthy benefits of high-fibre eating with good imaginative home cooking.

ENJOY SEX IN THE MIDDLE YEARS
Dr Christine Sandford

Dr Sandford gives plenty of sympathetic help on dealing with the worries that get in the way of a smooth, harmonious love life.

MIGRAINE AND HEADACHES
Dr Marcia Wilkinson

Migraine clinic Director Dr Marcia Wilkinson shows in this reassuring guide, how to cope with one of the commonest and often most distressing medical complaints.

GET A BETTER NIGHT'S SLEEP
Prof Ian Oswald & Dr Kirstine Adam

For the millions of insomniacs, these world-renowned sleep experts help to break the vicious circle of anxiety over lost sleep leading to more restless nights.

STRESS AND RELAXATION
Jane Madders

Jane Madders has developed her own simple techniques of natural relaxation that will help reduce stress in your everyday life.

New titles:

ACNE: ADVICE ON CLEARING YOUR SKIN
Prof Ronald Marks

A leading Professor of Dermatology tells you everything you need to know to help clear this condition that affects nearly all of us during teenage years and many into their twenties and beyond.

CONQUERING PAIN
Dr Sampson Lipton

Eminent pain-relief specialist Dr Sampson Lipton provides reliable and straightforward information to help you understand, avoid and overcome the pain.

EYES: THEIR PROBLEMS AND TREATMENTS
Michael Glasspool, FRCS

Many questions about common eye problems are answered in straightforward terms by Consultant Ophthalmic Surgeon Michael Glasspool.

OVERCOMING DYSLEXIA
Dr Bevé Hornsby

Dr Hornsby, a leading dyslexia specialist, answers your questions about one of today's most worrying and misunderstood conditions, which affects around one child in ten.